WHAT YOU MUST KNOW ABOUT
STATIN DRUGS
& THEIR NATURAL ALTERNATIVES

WHAT YOU MUST KNOW ABOUT
STATIN DRUGS
& THEIR NATURAL ALTERNATIVES

Jay S. Cohen, MD

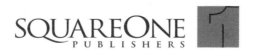

SQUAREONE
PUBLISHERS

The therapeutic procedures in this book are based on the training, personal experience, and research of the author. Because each person and situation is unique, the author and publisher urge the reader to check with a qualified health professional before using any procedure if there is any question to appropriateness.

The publisher does not advocate the use of any particular diet or health treatment, but believes the information presented in this book should be available to the public. Because there is always some risk involved, the author and publisher are not responsible for any adverse effects or consequences resulting from the use of any of the suggestions, preparations, or procedures described in this book. Please do not use the book if you are unwilling to assume the risk. Feel free to consult with a physician or other qualified health professional. It is a sign of wisdom, not cowardice, to seek a second or third opinion.

Cover Designer: Jacqueline Michelus
In-house Editors: Marie Caratozzolo and Elaine Weiser
Typesetters: Gary A. Rosenberg and Terry Wiscovitch

Square One Publishers
115 Herricks Road
Garden City Park, NY 11040
(516) 535-2010 • (877) 900-BOOK
www.squareonepublishers.com

Library of Congress Cataloging-in-Publication Data
Cohen, Jay S.
    What you must know about statin drugs & their natural alternatives : a consumer's guide to safely using lipitor, zocor, mevacor, crestor, pravachol, or natural alternatives / Jay S. Cohen.
        p. cm.
    Includes bibliographical references and index.
    ISBN 0-7570-0257-9 (pbk.)
    1. Statins (Cardiovascular agents)—Side effects—Popular works. 2. Hypercholesteremia— Alternative treatment—Popular works. I. Title.
RM666.S714C64   2005
615'.718—dc22
                                                                                    2004018904

Printed in the United States of America

10   9   8   7   6   5   4   3   2   1

Contents

Appendices

To Barbara and Rory

Acknowledgments

I love to learn, and I love writing and speaking about the things I have learned that may be of value to others for maintaining health and preventing or overcoming illness. Writing this book has been especially interesting because it has involved one of the most important and most controversial groups of medications available today: the statins. Thus, part of the fun of this project has been discussions I have had with respected mainstream doctors such as Dr. Ted Ganiats and Dr. Jeffrey Sandler, and with practitioners of complementary medicine such as Dr. Jeffrey Baker, Dr. Neil Hirschenbein, Dr. Ron Hoffman, Dr. Allan Magaziner, and Dr. Julian Whitaker. I would like to extend my appreciation to these and to the many other healthcare professionals who offered their perspectives.

Of course, a good idea, by itself, does not automatically become a book, so I want to thank Rudy Shur of Square One Publishers for his keen interest in this project and for his involvement and accessibility throughout the publishing process.

Finally, I would like to thank my family and friends for their unwavering support and encouragement of my work.

Preface

Good medical care requires good information. For the last fifteen years, I have been conducting independent research and publishing medical journal articles and consumer books to provide essential information to enable you and your doctor to use medications more safely and effectively than our current methods allow. This information is omitted from medication package inserts, the *Physicians' Desk Reference* (PDR), and doctors' and consumers' drug references.

My work on medication side effects and how to avoid them has gained considerable attention. I have been asked to write articles for national magazines and invited to speak at top-level medical conferences. In November 2002, for example, I was the keynote speaker at the Annual Science Day of the U.S. Food and Drug Administration, Clinical Pharmacology Division. I have also spoken at meetings of consumers, doctors, drug industry executives, and attorneys, and have debated the FDA's top medication expert on four different occasions, most recently in March 2004 at the conference of the American Society for Clinical Pharmacology and Therapeutics.

In addition, I have been on more than 100 radio shows across America, including National Public Radio. My research has been featured in virtually every major newspaper and magazine. My paper on the proper use of the antibiotics such as Cipro, used for treating anthrax, prompted the U.S. Centers for Disease Control to change their guidelines during the anthrax scare in 2001. Yet, despite this visibility, mainstream physicians have adopted few of my recommendations, and the problem of medication side effects—the fourth leading cause of death annually in America—continues unabated.

Why is this? One of the reasons that medication side effects remain a leading cause of death and disability year after year, decade after decade, is because important, independent information travels very slowly in the healthcare system. Drug companies control all of the major venues of information for doctors. This control is accomplished: by a sales force of 90,000 drug representatives who monitor doctors' prescribing patterns from pharmacy printouts and carry slanted information and freebies to doctors' offices on a weekly basis; by underwriting and influencing doctors' conferences and the majority of doctors' continuing education; by making the PDR, which is written by the drug industry, the book doctors use the most to guide their medication decisions; by possessing the vast majority of research money and filling medical journals with studies designed as much for marketing purposes as for medical progress; and by paying the salaries of more and more academicians at our medical schools, thereby focusing research and teaching on marketable drugs rather than on other issues of scientific importance.

The result is that for most disorders, treatment means drugs. Sometimes this is proper, sometimes not. The pharmaceutical industry's dominance over information also means that you are not likely to get a balanced viewpoint from most doctors today, because independent information about safer methods with medications and about scientifically-proven alternatives rarely reaches them. I have written *What You Must Know About Statin Drugs & Their Natural Alternatives* to fill this information void, so that you and your doctor can know all of the reasonable possibilities for reducing cholesterol, C-reactive protein, and other cardiovascular risk factors.

You have the right of informed consent with medications just as you do with surgery. Informed consent means receiving information about all of the treatments that may be effective for your condition. That is what this book provides: information about statin drugs and natural alternatives, and when and how to use them most effectively and safely.

What You Must Know About Statin Drugs & Their Natural Alternatives is written for people who:

- Have elevated cholesterol.

- Have an elevated C-reactive protein level.

- Have other known cardiovascular risk factors.

- Have had a heart attack or stroke.

- Are at risk of a heart attack, stroke, or atherosclerosis.

- Have a family history of cardiovascular disease.

- Are taking a statin medication.

- Have been given a prescription for a statin.

- Have heard about statins or have seen advertising on TV and wonder whether you might need a statin.

- Are having side effects with statins.

- Aren't getting satisfactory answers about side effects.

- Need treatment but don't like taking prescription drugs.

- Are interested in alternative methods instead of statins.

- Want to know about other strategies for preserving heart health.

- Want to know whether a low-fat or low-carbohydrate diet is best for you.

- Are concerned about family or friends taking statins.

- Want to save a lot on the high costs of statins.

- Want to minimize the risks of any treatment.

Medications help millions of people. Yet medication side effects harm millions more. Millions of other people discontinue vital treatment because of side effects or other dissatisfactions with current medical methods. These problems can be avoided. This book explains how to avoid them with statin medications and their natural alternatives. I hope you find this book informative and useful in attaining your health goals.

Jay S. Cohen, MD

WHAT YOU MUST KNOW ABOUT STATIN DRUGS
& THEIR NATURAL ALTERNATIVES

Introduction

How many of these questions about statin drugs, the top-selling drugs for lowering elevated levels of cholesterol and C-reactive protein, can you answer?

- Do I need to lower my cholesterol level?
- Do I need to take a statin drug?
- Which statin is best for me?
- What is the right dose for me?
- What are the side effects and how can I avoid them?
- Are there long-term risks with statins?
- If side effects occur, what can I do?
- Are there alternative methods I can use instead of statins?
- Are there other things I can do to preserve cardiovascular health?
- What is the best heart-healthy diet for me: low-carb or low-fat?
- How important is exercise, and how much is necessary?
- How can I save 50 percent or more off the high cost of statin drugs?

These are important questions for the 100 million Americans with elevated cholesterol. These questions are even more important for the 20 million Americans who take statin medications—Lipitor, Zocor, Pravachol, Mevacor, Lescol, or Crestor—and for the 25 million more who are slated to be taking statins soon.

Taking statins is simple, right? Elevated cholesterol = statins. Yet statins are potent drugs that can cause serious side effects. Are doctors prescribing statins with the care needed to use them effectively *and safely*? Are doctors carefully selecting the right statin at the right dose for people as individuals? Are doctors thinking about how to reduce people's risks of side effects and long-term toxicities? Are doctors offering you and others ways for keeping statin costs as low as possible? Are they informing you about other safer, proven-effective, less expensive alternatives? For many statin users today, the answer is no, no, no, no, and no.

Statins help millions of people, but like all drugs, they can also cause harm. Medicine's most respected pharmacology reference, *Goodman and Gilman's Pharmacological Basis of Therapeutics,* states: "Any drug, no matter how trivial its therapeutic actions, has the potential to do harm."[1] Statins' effects are not trivial.

Statins are very powerful chemicals that exert effects in every cell of your body. Many of these effects are good, but some can be bad. How can you maximize the benefits while minimizing the risks? Just as when buying a car or choosing a college for your child, the more information you have, the better your chances are of doing it right. What information do you need to take statins safely and effectively? That is what this book provides.

Most doctors will simply tell you that statins are safe and hand you a prescription. Yet statins have many common side effects that cause physical discomfort or mental impairment in millions of people. *Sixty to seventy-five percent of people started on statins stop taking them.*[2,3] *The average patient lasts only eight months on statins.*[3,4] Why? Side effects. Inadequate effects. Cost. These are the issues that come up again and again when I give seminars, speak with people, or read their letters. These are the problems that mainstream medicine has not learned to overcome.

But they can be overcome—indeed, they can be prevented—which is why I have written *What You Must Know About Statin Drugs & Their Natural Alternatives*. I am pro-medication and pro-statins, but my first responsibility, like all doctors, is to "Do No Harm." Sometimes doctors cannot avoid doing harm, but this is not the case with statin drugs. Statin risks can be dramatically reduced with a treatment model that emphasizes precision and safety, as this book will describe.

Statins can be very effective drugs—if given for the right reasons to the right persons at the right doses with the right treatment goals. Unfortunately, millions of people are prescribed statin doses that are too strong for their treatment goals, provoking side effects. Fifteen to forty-two percent of people given statins get side effects.[5-8] That's 7 to 15 million people. These side effects may be considered minor by doctors, but abdominal discomfort, muscle or joint pain, or memory impairment are not minor to you. And some statin side effects are not minor even to doctors: severe muscle pain or weakness, nerve injuries (some permanent), acute muscle breakdown, kidney and liver irritation or toxicity, and rarely, death.

Moreover, when 60 percent to 75 percent of people needing statins quit treatment, no one benefits. The long-term consequences of premature heart attacks and strokes harm not only patients and their families, but remain a costly, unsolved problem for hospitals, healthcare systems, insurers, and even the pharmaceutical industry and U.S. Food and Drug Administration.

The good news is that most of these problems are preventable, but only if you and your doctor know how. This is explained in Chapter 1, *Avoiding Statin Overtreatment or Undertreatment: The Precision-Prescribing, Safety-First Method.* The precision-prescribing, safety-first method will allow you to maximize the benefits of statins while minimizing the risks.

The most important question, of course, is whether you need statin therapy at all and, if so, how much? Chapter 2, *How Much Cholesterol Reduction Do You Really Need?*, answers these questions. Chapter 2 briefly explains the role of cholesterol, low density and high density-cholesterol (LDL-C, HDL-C), and C-reactive protein (CRP) on artery-clogging atherosclerosis and cardiac disease. Because of confusion about treatment goals, many doctors prescribe statin doses that are overly aggressive for people's requirements. This excessive treatment brings little extra benefit in exchange for significantly increased risks. It's not a good deal. That is why it is important for you and your doctor to know how much cholesterol-lowering is really beneficial, so treatment can be tailored to your needs and goals. Chapter 2 also tells you about five other risk factors that are often overlooked. These risk factors explain why half of the people who get heart attacks have normal cholesterol levels, so you want to know about them.

Chapter 3, *The Right Statin at the Right Dose*, explains why the standard initial doses of statins are unnecessarily strong for millions of people. Because of the omission of important information from package inserts and the *Physicians' Desk Reference* (PDR), many doctors, not intentionally, overshoot the mark when prescribing statins, giving patients very potent doses when mild ones would do. Chapter 3 describes who is most likely to benefit from the precision-prescribing method and what your goals should be when first starting treatment.

Chapter 4, *Low Dose Statins—The Evidence*, provides several strategies for choosing the right statin at the right dose for you. Chapter 4 presents the scientific evidence on the lower, safer, proven effective doses of each statin. It's not enough for me to say that lower statin doses work. Medical treatment should be based on scientific proof whenever possible, and that is what this chapter provides.

Chapter 5, *Why Do People Respond so Differently to Statin Drugs?*, explains why different people respond so differently to statin drugs. It explains why some people need strong statin doses while others need just a little, and how to identify each without causing harm. Chapter 6, *Women and Seniors—Special Considerations with Statin Drugs*, focuses on two groups that require extra attention and information in order to use statins effectively and safely. Few patients or their doctors know about the issues discussed in these chapters, but they are essential for optimal care with minimal risk.

Chapter 7, *Effective Strategies for Dealing with Side Effects and Other Problems with Statins*, answers the many questions that people sustaining statin side effects have asked me. Unfortunately, the medical system isn't very good about identifying or handling side effects, so I have divided Chapter 7 into seven sections that identify specific problems and offer practical solutions.

Many people do not like taking prescription drugs. If you're one of them, Chapter 8, *Effective Alternative Therapies for Reducing Cholesterol and Other Risk Factors*, is for you. There are several proven-effective alternative therapies worthy of consideration that cost much less than brand-name statins. Because making the right decisions about reducing cholesterol and other risk factors will have a major impact on your long-term health, I always recommend that you and your doctor make decisions about these alternative methods together.

Whether you take a statin or an alternative therapy or do nothing at all, there are four nutrients that everyone should consider for preventing cardiovascular disease. Chapter 9, *Essential Nutrients for Cardiovascular Health*, describes them and their importance: omega-3 fatty acids (fish oils), coenzyme Q_{10}, folic acid, and magnesium. Most people are sorely deficient in these nutrients, whose vital roles in maintaining a healthy heart and vascular system are backed by extensive scientific study.

Nutrition, of course, is also a big part of the equation for heart health. Yet there is so much confusion today. Low-carb or low-fat? Atkins or Ornish? Chapter 10, *Which Heart-Healthy Diet Is Right for You?*, provides original, clear guidelines to help you determine the best diet for you. This chapter also discusses exercise: the part it plays and the surprisingly little amount that's required to maintain heart health.

Obviously, you cannot take statins if you cannot afford them. Their high cost is another reason that people avoid taking statins, quit taking them, or take them less often than necessary. Chapter 11, *How to Cut Statin Costs by Fifty Percent or More*, explains why statin costs are so high and provides several strategies for substantially reducing the cost of treatment. This chapter also gives you a comparative analysis of statins versus natural alternatives, a cost analysis most doctors or healthcare systems have never seen or considered. If cost is an issue for you, you need to know about all of these options.

The book concludes with *Putting It All Together*, an overall strategy for setting your priorities and reaching your goals. Heart disease and strokes can be prevented. Vascular health can be preserved. By defining which steps you need—statin drugs or natural alternatives, essential nutrients, diet, and exercise—and how to easily employ them together, you and your doctor can decide how to improve the quality and extend the duration of your life.

I have written *What You Must Know About Statin Drugs & Their Natural Alternatives* to provide original, practical information that you will not find in statin package inserts, the PDR, or medical textbooks or consumer references on statins or medications. Most books on cholesterol discuss statins with the usual pharmaceutical industry slant, which is the information that results in millions of side effects and millions of people quitting needed treatment. Such methods are wasteful and harmful. *This book is much different: It is a primer on how you can decide whether you need treatment and, if so, exactly how much you need and how to accomplish it safely.*

The best treatment—statin or alternative—is the least powerful treatment that works. This book helps you define exactly what that is for you. In addition, unlike other books, this book provides information about essential nutrients that are vital, yet usually overlooked, for preserving cardiovascular health. Most doctors think they know everything they need to use statins properly, but they don't. I learned similar lessons the hard way when I treated patients. There is a tremendous amount of important information that doctors do not get through their usual sources, most of which comes from the pharmaceutical industry, and that you do not get through the media and typical bookstore references.

Most doctors and consumers do not know, for example, that medication side effects are the number four leading cause of death in America year after year, decade after decade. They also do not know that medication reactions cause more than 106,000 deaths, 1 million hospitalizations, and 2.2 million severe, often permanent disabilities each year.[9] Worse, these numbers may be underestimates because they represent only hospital patients, not the 100 million outpatients taking prescription drugs. Most doctors and consumers do not know that many of these problems are preventable. These problems can be prevented, but only if you and your doctor have the information needed for matching your treatment to your actual needs and tolerances. This is the basic principle of the precision-prescribing, safety-first method.

You have a right to information that makes it possible to obtain optimal care with minimum risk. This right is known as *informed consent*. This right applies to medication treatment just as it does to surgery. But to fully exercise your right of informed consent, you must receive enough information to make an intelligent choice. Most people do not receive enough information about statins to fully exercise their right of informed consent. Indeed, most people do not know that they have choices—many choices—about different doses and alternatives when considering statin drugs. Many of their doctors don't know this either. Unless you receive information about how to maximize the benefits while minimizing the risks and costs of statins, you have not received informed consent. You aren't alone. Studies show that only a small percentage of patients receive sufficient information to make an informed consent in doctors' offices.[10]

Statins can do a lot of good or cause serious harm. The difference depends on the decisions that are made based on the information available. The information available to most patients and their doctors today is inadequate to make informed choices for using statins safely and effectively. *What You Must Know About Statin Drugs & Their Natural Alternatives* provides the information you need to do just that.

1

Avoiding Statin Overtreatment or Undertreatment

The Precision-Prescribing, Safety-First Method

The statins are the most prescribed, most effective, and best tolerated of our cholesterol-lowering drugs. Some statins are household names. In 2001, Lipitor was the most prescribed drug in America, with patients filling 57,989,000 prescriptions at a cost of $5,223,784,000. Just behind was Zocor, third in sales at $3,679,839,000.[1] Pravachol, Mevacor, and Lescol remained brisk sellers as well, and Crestor's introduction to the pharmaceutical market in 2003 as the most powerful statin of all received considerable fanfare. Altogether, doctors wrote over 118 million prescriptions for statins in 2002. From March 2001 to 2003, statin sales jumped 32.5 percent, and Lipitor remained America's favorite prescription drug.[2] These numbers reflect the overwhelming confidence that most doctors have in statin drugs.

However, all of the advertising in the world would not make statins a top-selling group unless these drugs worked. Statins work by blocking a key step in the synthesis of cholesterol in the liver. The result is that statins reduce elevated cholesterol more effectively, with fewer side effects, than any other drugs. Statins also appear to reduce the inflammation—as measured by the C-reactive protein (CRP) level—that transforms bad cholesterol into atherosclerotic plaques that clog arteries. Studies have repeatedly proven that statins prevent the formation, slow the progression, and sometimes even cause the reversal of atherosclerosis. By doing so, statins reduce the incidence of coronary artery disease, heart attacks, strokes, and cardiac deaths by approximately 25 percent. So it is easy to see why mainstream doctors are bullish on statins, and why even alternative doctors sometimes use statins too.

PRECISION PRESCRIBING: DETERMINING THE RIGHT STATIN AT THE RIGHT DOSE FOR YOU

Statins are popular because they are powerful, but because they are powerful, they must be used properly. Statins are long-term drugs that must be taken year after year for decades in order to prevent heart attacks and strokes. Unfortunately, most people do not stick with statins very long. If you are to avoid being among the 60 percent to 75 percent who quit statin therapy prematurely, you must receive the right statin at the right dose for the right treatment goals.[3, 4] Too often today, people are prescribed statins that are too strong for their needs or tolerances. Side effects occur, which many doctors ignore, and people quit treatment. This is unfortunate, particularly because it is preventable.

How can you and your doctor maximize the benefits while minimizing the risks of statins? With the *precision-prescribing, safety-first method,* which ensures that you get the right statin at the right dose to achieve your goals. *Most problems with statins are not due to the drugs themselves, but are a result of the failure to tailor statin treatment to the individual.* Modern medicine is often shotgun medicine, in which drug companies and health providers are more concerned about treating large numbers of people than about individualizing treatment for your specific needs.

The result is that overtreatment and undertreatment occur very frequently with statin drugs. Overtreatment leads to side effects and people quitting treatment. Undertreatment causes inadequate cholesterol control and lack of benefit, and people quit treatment. The precision-prescribing method avoids both pitfalls. By carefully determining your proper statin drug and dose, the precision-prescribing method maximizes your chances of obtaining good cholesterol control while minimizing your risk of side effects.

STANDARD STARTING DOSES OF STATINS ARE NOT RIGHT FOR EVERYONE

Today, statins are prescribed to everyone in pretty much the same manner. The standard starting doses are set by the drug companies based on averaged responses from studies of thousands of patients. Most of these patients had heart disease and required strong cholesterol reductions. These averaged responses have led to the marketing of standard starting doses that are strong enough for some people, but too strong for many others.

Because these starting doses are recommended by the drug companies and approved by the FDA, these are the doses that most doctors prescribe when starting people on statins. Thus, the same strong initial statin doses are frequently prescribed to young and old, big and small, healthy and frail. These same strong initial doses are prescribed to people who take other medications and to people who don't. They are prescribed to people with a history of need-ing and tolerating strong medication doses and to those with a history of being very sensitive to medications or having a long list of medication reactions. This is cookbook medicine that treats everyone like a statistical average with its inevitably poor results. No wonder so many people quit statin therapy.

This situation is going to worsen with the release of two studies in which the highest dose of Lipitor, one of the strongest statins, slowed the develop-ment of plaque in arteries and reduced cardiac deaths more effectively than a moderate dose of moderate-strength Pravachol.[5,6] Based on these results in a very select group of patients with acute coronary disease, some doctors began using much stronger statin therapy for almost anyone with elevated cholesterol. In July 2004, the American Heart Association and other experts released new, lower target cholesterol guidelines for people at high risk for heart disease. This has led to the increased use of the stronger statins at stronger doses, even for people who require only modest cholesterol reduc-tions that can be accomplished with dietary measures, lower statin doses, or natural alternatives. Indeed, some doctors are starting patients at doses stronger than those recommended by the drug companies themselves. But millions of people with elevated cholesterol do not need such extreme ther-apy, and even those who do will not necessarily tolerate super-strong statin doses from the start. The incidence and severity of statin side effects is going to rise even higher, and we will soon read about terrible reactions to these drugs that will scare everyone. This is an undesirable, avoidable situation. There is a better way of getting people to their treatment goals.

EMPHASIZING SAFETY WITH STATINS

The precision-prescribing method considers factors such as your age, size, gender, state of health, and whether you are taking other medications. It considers whether you have a history of side effects with medications or display other signs of medication or chemical intolerances, or whether you may be a fast metabolizer who tends to metabolize medications quickly and requires stronger doses than the average person.

The precision-prescribing method places an emphasis on preventing side effects. It places an emphasis on initiating treatment in an individual-ized manner with a statin drug and dose that are not too strong for you: A start-low, go-slow approach. The precision-prescribing method is based on the belief that keeping people in treatment long-term is more important than initiating treatment aggressively. Reducing cholesterol usually is not an emergency. Successful statin therapy requires a long-term strategy, not an immediate, high-risk intervention. Successful therapy requires the recognition that treatment is a marathon, not a sprint.

The precision-prescribing model encourages a flexible approach to starting treatment with statins. It recommends gradual, stepwise tactics toward reaching your treatment goals. By emphasizing safety, the precision-prescribing method focuses on preventing overmedication and the avoidable side effects it causes. By initiating treatment gradually and comfortably—starting low, going slow—side effects will not drive you from treatment. Quite the contrary: because the precision-prescribing method employs a stepwise approach, you can be sure that if the initial dose does not accomplish your treatment goals, subsequent careful increases in dosage will. You can be sure that you will never get more medication than you actually need, with its higher risk of side effects, yet undertreatment will also be avoided.

THE PROBLEM WITH THE MAINSTREAM "MIDDLE-DOSE" APPROACH

The precision-prescribing method offers an alternative model for using statins that stands in stark contrast to the "middle-dose approach" sanctioned by the drug industry and FDA. Their middle-dose approach endorses the use of strong initial doses to cover populations of hundreds of millions of people. Fearing undertreatment that will discourage doctors and patients, the middle-dose approach leads to the overtreatment of millions. At the same time, the middle-dose approach allows drug companies to ignore lower doses that would complicate their marketing plans, despite the fact that these lower, safer doses were proven effective in their own research. By quashing information about these lower doses that work for millions of patients, the middle-dose approach guarantees that with standard doses, these people will receive 100 percent to 400 percent more medication than they actually need. This overmedication provokes a predictable avalanche of side effects—preventable side effects—that make people miserable, disrupt treatment, and explain why the statistics on side effects and treatment adherence are so poor.

What is the attitude of the middle-dose proponents regarding side effects? They advise that when side effects occur, then the dosage should be lowered. What a comforting idea! After you have suffered muscle pain or

Individual Variation and Drug Doses

Medical experts agree that people vary greatly in their responses to medications and that using the lowest effective doses is the key to avoiding medication side effects.

■ **U.S. Food and Drug Administration:** "Historically, drugs have often been initially marketed at what were later recognized as excessive doses. . . . Any given dose provides a mixture of desirable and undesirable effects, with no single dose necessarily optimal for all patients."[22]

■ *Goodman and Gilman's Pharmacologic Basis of Therapeutics:* "Therapy as a science does not apply simply to the evaluation and testing of new, investigational drugs in animals and man. It applies with equal importance to the treatment of each patient as an individual."[23]

■ *Goth's Medical Pharmacology:* "A perplexing problem for both pharmacologists and physicians is the variation that occurs among normal subjects as well as among patients in response to a particular drug. This individual variability necessitates a correspondingly wide range of doses among patients."[7]

■ **American Medical Association Drug Evaluations:** "Almost all drugs cause reasonably predictable toxic reactions when given in excessive doses."[18]

■ *British Medical Journal (BMJ):* "Many drugs have been introduced at doses that later were found to be too high; and usually years have passed, with unnecessary toxicity, before action was taken."[25]

abdominal discomfort or memory problems, then your doctor will finally consider adjusting the statin dose according to your individual needs. Isn't this backward? What a wasteful, risky model! And you are the one placed at risk. In fact, not all side effects are reversible. Muscle breakdown, kidney injuries, and liver toxicities are not easily repaired. When the middle-dose approach was used with the statin Baycol, dozens of deaths occurred and the drug was ultimately withdrawn after the fact. Baycol victims did not get an opportunity to the try lower, safer, proven-effective doses of Baycol that should have been prescribed for many of them in the first place.

The reality is that the middle-dose approach is contrary to patients' desire for safety and doctors' credo of "Do No Harm." Nevertheless, the middle-dose approach is currently the authorized approach of the drug industry and FDA, and it is reflected in the standard starting doses of scores of drugs that are double or quadruple the strength that millions of people need. I have debated the wisdom of the middle-dose approach at major medical conferences and at the FDA itself. They acknowledge my point, but so far little has changed.

AVOIDING OVERTREATMENT AND UNDERTREATMENT

Many adverse reactions arise from failure to tailor the dosage of drugs to widely different individual needs.[7]
—GOTH'S MEDICAL PHARMACOLOGY

In contrast to the middle-dose approach, the precision-prescribing method emphasizes the need to prevent side effects by matching statin doses to the individual. It emphasizes a start-low go-slow approach that starts treatment at a low, proven-effective dose before going to higher, stronger, riskier doses of these powerful drugs. By avoiding the excessive dosing that is so prevelant with statins today, common side effects are avoided and long-term risks are minimized. By involving you in the process, this approach guards against the undertreatment that fails to produce results and discourages and alienates patients.

The precision-prescribing method is new for statins, but not new in the realm of medicine. Smart doctors employ a similar method with drugs for hypertension (high blood pressure), because these drugs have many side effects that drive millions of people from vital treatment. That's why experts recommend starting low and going slow with antihypertensive drugs. The precision-prescribing method is also the state of the art with insulin and thyroid medications, where precision is essential or people very quickly develop serious side effects. Unfortunately, the great majority of medications are not prescribed with such precision. One-size-fits-all dosing is common today. More and more drugs are released with fewer and fewer dosage options. Many drugs are prescribed at the same potent doses for the young and old, big and small, healthy and frail. Most of these drugs could be prescribed via the precision-prescribing, start-low go-slow model. They should be. And statins are the foremost example.

Millions of people need statins, but the question is: How much is enough? If you need Zocor, should your doctor start with the drug company–recommended initial doses of 20 mg or 40 mg, or just 5 mg? Or with Lipitor, the original drug company–recommended initial dose of 10 mg, or newly approved initial doses of 20 or 40 mg, or just 2.5 mg? The same question applies to all statin drugs. Should you begin with a standard middle-dose or with a lower, safer, proven effective dose? This is the key decision, because although many people do well on statins, many people do not. Statins may be good drugs, but like all drugs, they are potent foreign chemicals that can cause side effects and often do, so overtreatment is something you want to avoid.

Healthcare systems also play a role in the overtreatment and undertreatment with statins. By influencing doctors to keep patients' visits few, these healthcare systems discourage a careful, stepwise, start-low go-slow approach that requires follow-up in order to arrive at your proper statin dose as safely as possible. This causes doctors to prescribe strong doses to make sure that patients get adequate cholesterol reductions, a shotgun approach that results in the overmedication of millions of people. At the same time, these standard doses are not enough for people requiring even stronger statin therapy, causing the undertreatment of millions more.

Undertreatment should never occur with statins because it is so easily avoided. Once you start on a statin, you are supposed to return for follow-up visits to ensure that you have reached your treatment goals. If the initial statin dose does not reduce your cholesterol levels enough, it should be increased gradually until your goals are reached. It's that simple. Thus, when undertreatment occurs, it is usually due to a failure of the system to provide adequate follow-up or of patients failing to keep follow-up appointments, not of the statin itself. Sometimes, however, when statin doses are increased, side effects occur. This is because statin doses are sometimes increased in 100 percent jumps that are too strong for many people (see Chapter 4).

Overtreatment occurs more commonly than undertreatment and has more serious consequences. Approximately 15 to 40 percent of people taking statins get side effects, usually as abdominal discomfort, muscle or joint pain, muscle weakness, memory problems, or liver irritation.[8–11] In one analysis, 65 percent of patients taking Lipitor reported side effects.[12] Moreover, in rare cases, statins have caused death from acute muscle degeneration or liver toxicity. There have also been thousands of reports of serious cognitive and psychiatric problems that do not always disappear when statins are discontinued. And now we are hearing about nerve injuries, sometimes severe and permanent, with long-term statin use. All of this will worsen as doctors push stronger statins indiscriminately. Even in the recent landmark studies, strong-dose Lipitor caused significantly more side effects than moderate-dose Pravachol, yet doctors, readily exclaiming their delight with the positive aspects of the studies, ignored this issue entirely.

THE DOSE MAKES THE DIFFERENCE

The key to avoiding such side effects with statins is to treat people as individuals by determining the right dose with the least risk from the start. Avoiding overmedication is key because most statin side effects are *dose-related*. Higher doses may work more quickly to reduce cholesterol levels, but unless you actually need a higher dose, all you get is their greater risks.[10–14] For example, the risk of liver injury from excessive statin doses has been quantified. Dr. W. C. Roberts, the editor-in-chief of the *American Journal of Cardiology*, warns: "With each doubling of the dose, the frequency of liver enzyme elevations [indicating liver irritation or injury] also doubles."[13]

The American Heart Association states that liver enzyme elevations occur in 1 percent to 2 percent of people taking statins. With 40 million people slated to take statins, that's 400,000 to 800,000 people. Elevated liver enzymes, if ignored, can lead to liver damage. Liver toxicity and, rarely, death from liver failure have been reported with statins. The American Heart Association advises that a reduction in liver enzyme levels "is frequently noted with a reduction in dose."[15] In other words, the way to avoid these problems is to use the lowest statin dose each person needs, not the highest dose that makes treating a lot of people convenient for a fast-paced healthcare system.

Statins are not unique in this regard: side effects with most drugs are dose-related. Experts estimate that 75 percent to 80 percent of all medication side effects are dose-related.[16,17] Actually, the number is even higher, because drug interactions are also more frequent and severe when people receive higher doses of drugs. When you add these together, it reveals that 85 percent to 90 percent of all side effects may be dose-related. When you consider that medication side effects are the fourth leading cause of death in the U.S., causing more than 100,000 deaths and millions of severe reactions annually, according to the *Journal of the American Medical Association (JAMA)*, and that these problems occur at the standard doses that drug companies recommend and doctors routinely prescribe, the importance of using the lowest, safest drug doses for each person becomes even more obvious. That is why the precision-prescribing, safety-first model works so well, because it does just that.

INDIVIDUAL VARIATION: THE FORGOTTEN FACTOR

The dose-related nature of drug effects is obvious in everyday life: the more coffee you drink, the greater the likelihood of edginess or insomnia; the more alcohol, the greater the impairment of coordination or judgment. Individual sensitivity also plays a role. Some people are sensitive to the effects of chemical agents while others are not. Some people can handle a pot of coffee, while others can't handle a cup. Some people can tolerate high doses of statins, while others get adverse effects at modest doses. This really is not surprising: a basic principle of medical science is *inter-individual variation*, the wide range of variation between people in response to the same drugs at the same doses.

Individual variation with drugs is not the exception, it is the rule. Indeed, the American Medical Association states that the difference in people's response to a drug can vary "4- to 40-fold."[18] This is why some people get large cholesterol reductions with low statin doses, while others require large statin doses to get modest reductions. And why some people are so sensitive to statin drugs they tolerate only tiny statin doses. Thus, the two keys to understanding side effects and how to avoid them are:

1. Because the great majority of side effects are dose-related, the best dose is the least amount that works for you.

2. Individuals vary greatly in their responses to drugs. Some people require high-dose statins, others low-dose statins, and others something in between. To avoid excessive dosing, doses must be tailored for each person based on his or her treatment goals and sensitivity to statin effects.

The precision-prescribing method is predicated on these fundamental medical principles. The middle-dose, mass-marketing methods of the drug industry and FDA ignore these principles, and the result is an epidemic of side effects—dose-related side effects. My belief is that any side effect that is dose-related can be avoided by starting low and going slow—by emphasizing safety first. Most patients agree with me. When I treated patients from 1971 to 1990, I often gave them a choice: starting with a standard drug-company middle dose or with a lower, proven-effective dose. Eighty percent or more chose the latter, and successful treatment, sticking with treatment, and patient satisfaction all rose to unprecedented levels.

EXCESSIVE DOSING PROVOKES UNNECESSARY SIDE EFFECTS

Duane Graveline is a retired family doctor, flight surgeon, and astronaut. Prescribed Lipitor by his own doctor, Dr. Graveline developed amnesia "so severe that I landed in the emergency room of a hospital near my Vermont home. I didn't remember any of it."

Amnesia is not the cute little memory loss depicted by Hollywood. It is a dangerous, frightening experience. For twelve hours, Dr. Graveline was never a doctor, never an astronaut, never married, and did not recognize his wife when she found him wandering aimlessly in the woods behind his house. Imagine the consequences if Dr. Graveline had been driving. Like his memory, all of his mechanical skills had abruptly vanished as well.

Dr. Graveline was perplexed by his reaction. After all, he was not usually sensitive to medications, and he had taken only 10 mg, the lowest dose recommended and marketed by the manufacturer. Yet 10 mg of Lipitor is quite strong, much stronger than many people need. It was much stronger than Dr. Graveline needed, because he needed only 2.5 mg of Lipitor—¼ the dose that he was prescribed.

How do I know how much Lipitor Dr. Graveline should have received? Because the guidelines are clear. Experts advise doctors to select statin doses based on the reduction in LDL-C and overall cardiovascular risk.[19] For example, the American Society of Health-System Pharmacists advises: "Dosage of statins must be carefully adjusted according to individual requirements and response."[8] Ten milligrams of Lipitor reduces LDL-C 39 percent,[9] a strong response needed by cardiac patients or people with severely elevated cholesterol or multiple risk factors. But most people with high cholesterol have mild to moderate elevations and no cardiac history, and they usually require LDL-C reductions of only 20 percent to 30 percent. Although you will not find a word about it in statin package inserts, the PDR,[9] or other drug references, studies show that these reductions can be obtained with only 2.5 or 5 mg of Lipitor.

Dr. Graveline required a 25 percent reduction in LDL-C, so he should have been started with 2.5 mg of Lipitor. Yet the smallest Lipitor pill is 10 mg, and because there's no information about 2.5 or 5 mg of Lipitor in the package insert or PDR, many people are started at this dose. Some people are started at 20 or 40 mg of Lipitor. Now some doctors are suggesting that 80 mg of Lipitor is the best amount. Imagine what would have happened if Dr. Graveline received this dose initially. When drug companies do not provide information about the lowest, safest, effective doses, such as 2.5 and 5 mg of Lipitor, it makes safe, individualized treatment impossible and causes side effects that could, and should, be avoided.

PREVENTING SIDE EFFECTS: AN URGENT HEALTHCARE ISSUE

Most doctors follow the drug companies' guidelines for prescribing medications, including statins. These guidelines are listed in the "Dosage and

Administration" sections of package inserts and the PDR, which is a compendium of package inserts. If you compare the initial doses recommended in the PDR to doses in studies published in the medical literature, you will see that the drug company-recommended initial doses of many drugs, including statins, are stronger than many people need. This is a result of the pharmaceutical industry's and FDA's adherence to the middle-dose approach. I have written a dozen papers in leading medical journals and two books on this issue, pointing out that we could greatly reduce the incidence of side effects by starting patients with lower, safer medication doses that have already been proven effective in scores of scientific studies. For many people, these lower doses work fine and never need to be raised.

Preventing side effects is an urgent healthcare issue. As the statistics presented previously show, the incidence of side effects is at epidemic proportions. It has been that way for decades and will continue to be until we adopt better, safer methods. As the researchers of the study that defined the scope of the side-effect epidemic concluded: "The incidence of serious and fatal adverse drug reactions in U.S. hospitals was found to be extremely high."[16] And if you add the millions of medication reactions in outpatients, the numbers are even higher. Most important, these side effects occur at the same doses that drug companies recommend and the FDA approves. The researchers underscored this fact: "There are a large number of serious adverse drug reactions even when the drugs are properly prescribed and administered."[16]

Obviously, the "proper doses" are not so proper for millions of people. My research has gone a step further and explained, (as I wrote in 2000): "Our ongoing epidemic of side effects is in large part the result of so-called standard doses that are too strong for large segments of the population."[20]

In other words, the side-effect epidemic is the consequence of the drug companies' and FDA's adherence to the shotgun, middle-dose approach that is designed for treating broad populations rather than ensuring that you get the right amount of medication for you. By emphasizing mass marketing over individual safety, the result is inevitable: millions of toxicities that could and should be prevented.

I readily acknowledge that medications are one of our foremost healing tools. Forty-six percent of all Americans benefit from a prescription drug everyday; many millions more benefit from the intermittent use of prescription or over-the-counter drugs. Moreover, medications have played a significant role in the 40 percent increase in longevity from 1900 to 2000, when the average lifespan increased from 47 to 76 years. I am pro-medication when medications are used properly.

But I am also a hawk about minimizing your risk. Doctors are supposed to try to "Do No Harm," but how can doctors do so in a system that guarantees tremendous harm—preventable harm? With statins, a backlash is already developing because of the shotgun, expedient methods of mainstream medicine. Recently, *The Wall Street Journal* reported:

> There is a quiet backlash brewing against statins. . . . A number of critics believe drug companies have vastly understated side effects caused by statins—particularly muscle pains and memory problems. As a result, when patients complain of muscle aches and fuzzy thinking, many doctors don't even consider that a statin might be the culprit, and instead just assume the patient is getting old like the rest of us. Drug companies maintain that side effects are rare, and that the benefits of statins far outweigh any risk.[21]

Denial by doctors and drug companies will not solve the problem. It is only making things worse. Yet the problem can be readily solved by using statins safely based on individual needs and tolerances. Precision-prescribing should not be reserved for insulin and thyroid drugs and a few others. It can be applied to most drugs. By doing so, the benefits you obtain from statins can be maximized, while the risks are minimized. Accomplishing this requires information about statin drugs that you will not get from package inserts, the PDR, references in doctors' offices, or on bookstore shelves. Accomplishing this depends on a precision-prescribing, start-low, go-slow approach based on your statin sensitivity and on how much cholesterol-lowering you actually need.

2

How Much Cholesterol Reduction Do You Really Need?

The Essentials on LDL-C, HDL-C, C-Reactive Protein, and Other Important Risk Factors

Of all the common causes of premature death—heart attack, stroke, cancer, accidents, diabetes, and infections diseases—the odds are greatest that you are going to die from a heart attack or stroke. This is true whether you are male or female.[1]

—ARTEMIS SIMOPOULOS, MD, FORMER CHAIRMAN OF THE
NUTRITION COORDINATING COMMITTEE OF THE NATIONAL
INSTITUTES OF HEALTH

Each year, nearly 1 million Americans—over 2,500 a day, 100 an hour—die from cardiovascular disease, and 6 million are hospitalized. Each year, heart disease is our number one cause of death in men and women, and strokes are number three. Cardiovascular disease costs the American economy an estimated $274 billion annually. But this is not just an American problem: overall, about 45 percent of adults in western societies die from cardiovascular disease.[2]

Most people are aware of the importance of maintaining cardiovascular health, but as more and more information emerges and the theories and guidelines keep changing, many people, including doctors, are confused. How can you prevent cardiovascular disease and maintain a healthy heart and blood vessels? How can you prevent a heart attack or stroke? What are the most important risk factors? What is the best approach? These are important questions, yet the answers keep changing as we identify new risk factors and redefine factors already recognized. Moreover, different experts interpret the information differently. When it comes down to receiving statin therapy, the basics are pretty well defined, and the choice of the drug and dose you receive should be based on the amount of reduction in cholesterol you require and other risk factors you may have.

THE IMPORTANCE OF REDUCING LOW-DENSITY LIPOPROTEIN CHOLESTEROL (LDL-C)

Atherosclerosis underlies most cardiovascular disease. It is the development of plaques in arteries from accumulations of cholesterol combined with fatty droplets, platelets, and inflammatory cells. Atherosclerotic plaques can enlarge and block arteries to the heart, brain, kidneys, or limbs. Or the plaques can rupture, spewing their contents into arteries and triggering artery-blocking clots.

The body manufactures cholesterol for a reason. Cholesterol is an important component of healthy cells and essential for normal body functioning. Cholesterol is needed for building cell membranes; producing hormones such as estrogen, testosterone, and cortisol; and as a component of bile, which helps clear toxins from the body. But excess cholesterol can be a killer. Since 1993, studies have repeatedly shown that lowering elevated cholesterol levels reduces coronary disease, heart attacks, and cardiac deaths.[4–8] That is why mainstream experts now recommend statin drugs for 35 million Americans with elevated cholesterol levels.[9] Most alternative doctors I know agree about the role of cholesterol in cardiovascular disease. "Your body is capable of producing all the cholesterol it needs, so there's no need to eat a lot of cholesterol," states Dr. Julian Whitaker, one of America's best-known alternative physicians. "Excess cholesterol that isn't eliminated from your body is likely to be deposited in the walls of arteries, causing them to narrow and stiffen."[3] The result: cardiovascular mayhem—blocked arteries, heart attacks, strokes, reduced circulation to the kidneys and limbs.

Because cholesterol is not water soluble, it must be transported in the bloodstream. This is accomplished by linking with protein-fat substances called lipoproteins. You're probably already familiar with LDL-C and HDL-C, the acronyms for low-density lipoprotein cholesterol and high-density lipoprotein cholesterol (see the inset on page 21). Lowering cholesterol usually means lowering LDL-cholesterol, the bad low-density lipoprotein cholesterol that is closely linked with atherosclerosis. The highly respected National Cholesterol Education Program (Adult Treatment Panel III) (NCEP, for short) states:

> Research from experimental animals, laboratory investigations, epidemiology, and genetic forms of hypercholesterolemia [high blood cholesterol] indicate that elevated LDL cholesterol is a major cause of coronary heart disease. In addition, recent clinical trials robustly show that LDL-lowering therapy reduces the risk for coronary heart disease.[10]

How important is it to reduce LDL-cholesterol? The risk of coronary disease is directly correlated with people's levels of LDL-C.[11] For example, people with coronary disease whose LDL-C levels are elevated have a twelve-fold greater likelihood of dying from a heart attack than people whose LDL-C levels are normal.[12] Reducing high LDL-C levels directly reduces cardiac risk. How much? The American Society of Hospital Pharmacists reports:

> It has been estimated that each 1% reduction in LDL cholesterol may result in a 1% decrease in the incidence of coronary heart disease.[13]

BENEFITS OF HIGH-DENSITY LIPOPROTEIN CHOLESTEROL (HDL-C)

A high level of the good HDL-cholesterol can partially offset the risk of a high LDL-C. The higher your HDL-C level, the lower your cardiac risk. Even if your LDL-C is very low (below 100 mg/dl), you still have a greater risk of heart disease if your HDL-C is low. Indeed, some studies suggest that HDL-C levels may be as important or an even more important indicator of cardiac risk than LDL-C. This appears to be especially true for women. Moreover, new studies using experimental drugs that enhance HDL-C have demonstrated the ability to reverse atherosclerosis somewhat.

Experts recommend a HDL-C level of at least 45 mg/dl for men and 55 mg/dl for women. Some people have much higher HDL-C levels, but others have great difficulty reaching these levels because HDL-C levels are

---

Types of Cholesterol

TC = Total Cholesterol: The total amount of cholesterol in the blood measured in mg/dl (milligrams per deciliter). Your total cholesterol level is comprised of HDL-C, LDL-C, and VLDL-C.

HDL-C = High-Density Lipoprotein Cholesterol: The good cholesterol that protects against atherosclerosis. High HDL-C levels indicate a reduced risk of cardiovascular disease.

LDL-C = Low-Density Lipoprotein Cholesterol: The bad cholesterol, linked to increased heart attacks, strokes, and sudden cardiac death. Lowering LDL-C reduces the risk. LDL-C is the key level in determining the types of treatment.

VLDL-C = Very Low-Density Lipoprotein Cholesterol: Another type of bad cholesterol, usually present in much smaller amounts than LDL-C.

genetically determined to a large degree. Exercise and the consumption of good oils (e.g., olive, canola) can elevate HDL-C levels modestly.

DO YOU NEED TO LOWER YOUR CHOLESTEROL LEVEL?

If you are one of the 42 million Americans with cholesterol levels above 240 mg/dl, you need to lower it. But this needn't always mean prescription drugs. Today, many doctors—alternative and mainstream—are questioning whether more and more drugs are the answer for everyone with elevated LDL-C. And a few scientists question whether cholesterol is really the primary culprit in atherosclerosis in the first place. Most people aren't interested in these academic debates. They just want to know what to do. If your LDL-C is elevated, you have several choices: dietary management, prescription drugs, or natural alternatives. These choices are not mutually exclusive, and no matter which other approaches you use, a heart-healthy diet is always number one. But if a good diet is not enough, how do you decide what to do next? First, it depends on which group you are in:

Primary Prevention Group: People with no history of cardiovascular disease, but with high cholesterol. The goal here is purely preventive.

Secondary Prevention Group: People with cardiovascular disease and high cholesterol, for whom the goal is to prevent further damage by reducing cholesterol to much lower levels.

   The current guidelines for optimal cholesterol and LDL-C levels are listed on pages 24–25. The vast majority of people with elevated LDL-C are in the low- or moderate-risk groups. If you are in the low-risk group and have moderately elevated cholesterol and few other risk factors, your target LDL-C is 160 mg/dl, although a level of 130 is considered better. For this group, a heart-healthy diet is the first and best choice. Beyond this, doctors disagree. Some prescribe statins, but others argue that the risks and costs of statins are not worth the small gains in this group, especially for people without family histories of heart attacks or strokes.

   If you are in the primary prevention group and have very high LDL-C levels, or multiple risk factors such as hypertension (even if it is being treated) or a family history of early cardiovascular disease, your target LDL-C is 130. Some experts recommend a target of 100 or lower. Treatment goals and methods vary based on your number of risk factors and other risk indicators, as detailed on pages 24–25.

   If you are in the secondary prevention group, you have cardiovascular disease and are therefore high risk. Preventing further damage is impera- tive. Mortality is high for people who survive a first heart attack but do not receive ongoing treatment: 5 percent mortality a year with a cumulative car- diovascular mortality of 70 percent after fifteen years. After a second heart attack, cardiovascular mortality is 10 percent per year without consistent treatment. "The high mortality rate emphasizes the need to ensure that everyone who has had an MI (heart attack), even years previously, receives effective preventive treatment," an article in the *Archives of Internal Medicine* advised.[14] Thus, the LDL-C goal in the secondary prevention group is lower than in the primary prevention group: below 100 mg/dl or even lower.

In a study of 4,162 patients hospitalized for acute chest pain from heart disease, some of these "acute coronary syndrome" patients received a mod- erate 40 mg dose of Pravachol, which was strong enough to produce an LDL-C of 95 mg/dl on average—the target level based on current guide- lines. Other patients received the strongest dose of Lipitor, 80 mg, dropping their LDL-C level to 62 mg/dl on average. Within a month, the Lipitor group was already demonstrating greater benefits than the Pravachol group. After two years, the number of people in the Pravachol group requir- ing angioplasty or bypass surgery, or experiencing chest pain, heart attack, stroke, or death was 26.3 percent as compared with 22.4 percent of those on Lipitor.[15] Based on this and other recent studies, experts have lowered the target LDL-C levels for these very high-risk patients to less than 70 mg/dl.

No matter which group you are in, unless you are in an acute risk cat- egory, precision-prescribing is always the best approach, because some peo- ple obtain major cholesterol reductions with low or moderate statin doses and because precision-prescribing is the best way to minimize drug risks and satisfy patients' concerns about side effects. Indeed, in the Pravachol- Lipitor study mentioned above, patients' liver enzymes were elevated in 1.1 percent of Pravachol users versus 3.3 percent of those on Lipitor—a huge difference. That is 33,000 people for every million taking high-dose Lipitor compared with 11,000 people for every million taking moderate-dose Pravachol—in other words, 22,000 more people with adverse liver effects for every million taking super-strong Lipitor, and some of these liver injuries will be serious. We should also remember that when the statin Bay- col was withdrawn in 2001 because of deaths in patients, most of these peo- ple were taking the strongest Baycol dose.

Some doctors recognize this. Many others do not. Some doctors are appro- priately cautious about who requires aggressive treatment and how aggres- sively to initiate it. Others prescribe aggressive therapy for everyone. You need

Your Risk Category and LDL-C Lowering Requirement

There are four risk categories: low, moderate, moderate-high, and high risk. In order to find your category, you need to determine how many risk factors you have. Risk factors include (add 1 risk factor for each that you have): Age (males over 44, females over 54); high blood pressure (even if being treated); cigarette smoking; a family history of early coronary disease; an HDL level below 40 mg/dl. If your HDL level is 60 or higher, you can subtract one risk factor.

Low-Risk Category: You are in this category if you have 0 or 1 risk factors and do not have cardiovascular disease or diabetes. Your goal is an LDL-C level below 160 mg/dl (some experts recommend an LDL-C below 130).

- If your LDL-C is between 160 and 189: you should initiate diet and other lifestyle changes.*
- If your LDL-C is 190 or higher: you should initiate diet and other lifestyle changes. If these do not reduce your LDL-C below 160, medication or alternative therapy should be considered.

Moderate-Risk Category: You are in this category if you have 2 or more risk factors, but you do not have cardiovascular disease or diabetes, and other risk indicators are few.** Your goal is an LDL-C level below 130 mg/dl.

- If your LDL-C is 130 to 159, you should initiate diet and lifestyle changes.
- If your LDL-C is 160 or higher: you should initiate diet and other lifestyle changes. If these do not reduce your LDL-C below 130, medication or alternative therapy should be considered.

Moderate-High-Risk Category: You are in this category if you do not have cardiovascular disease or diabetes, but you have 2 or more risk factors and your other risk indicators are considerable.** Your goal is an LDL-C level below 130 mg/dl, although some experts recommend an LDL-C below 100.

- If your LDL-C is 130 or higher: initiate diet and lifestyle changes. If these do not reduce your LDL-C below 130, medication therapy should be considered. The same guidelines apply if you and your doctor decide that your goal is an LDL-C below 100, and your current LDL-C is 100 or above.
- No matter what your LDL-C level is, you should initiate diet and lifestyle changes if you: are overweight by 20 pounds or more; are physically inactive; have an elevated triglyceride level; or your HDL-C is below 40; or have metabolic syndrome (see Chapter 10).

High-Risk Category: You are in the high-risk category if you have heart or other atherosclerotic vascular disease, diabetes, or other factors that indicate a very high degree of risk.** The goal for this category is an LDL-C below 100 mg/dl. However, for people with advanced cardiovascular disease or diabetes, or who are otherwise considered at very high risk, an LDL-C below 70 mg/dl is preferable.

- If your LDL-C is 100 or higher: You should initiate diet and other lifestyle changes as well as medication therapy. The same guidelines apply if you and your doctor decide that your goal is a LDL-C below 70, and your current LDL-C is above this number.
- No matter what your LDL-C level is, you should initiate diet and lifestyle changes if you: are overweight by 20 pounds or more; are physically inactive; have an elevated triglyceride level; or your HDL-C is below 40; or you have metabolic syndrome (see Chapter 10).

*Lifestyle changes include regular moderate exercise, maintaining a healthy weight, not smoking, and stress reduction. Initiating dietary and other lifestyle changes are very important because they can reduce your cardiovascular risk via several mechanisms, in addition to lowering your LDL C.

**The measurement of cardiovascular risk sometimes involves a second, complicated calculation that assesses risk factors more closely. The best way to obtain this calculation is via the American Heart Association's program at: http://www.americanheart.org/presenter.jhtml?identifier=3003499.

This information is adapted from the 2004 guidelines from the National Cholesterol Education Program.[35]

to decide how you want your treatment to be conducted. With the information in this book, you can take an active part with your doctor in doing so.

C-REACTIVE PROTEIN: THE NEW RISK FACTOR

Half of all cardiac deaths occur in people with normal cholesterol levels. Clearly, other factors are involved. New studies suggest that an elevated level of C-reactive protein (CRP), an indicator of inflammation, may be as important an indicator of cardiac risk as cholesterol levels.[16,17] In fact, emerging evidence suggests that an elevated CRP may also be an indicator of an increased risk of high blood pressure, colon cancer, Alzheimer's disease, and perhaps many other disorders.

C-reactive protein is produced in the liver and other tissues in response to infection or inflammation anywhere in the body. CRP is manufactured as part of the body's immune response against infection and injury, but this immune response can cause damage if it produces excess inflammation in a person's own tissues. For years, experts have suspected that inflammation in artery walls played an important role in causing atherosclerosis—and in other diseases, too. "Forward-thinking cardiologists now suspect that internal inflammation is the root cause of many diseases including those of the heart and blood vessels," states cardiologist Dr. Stephen Sinatra.[18]

It is now believed that millions of Americans with elevated CRP are at risk even though their cholesterol levels are normal. Dr. Paul Ridker, Director of the Center for Cardiovascular Disease Prevention at Brigham and Women's Hospital in Boston, told *The New York Times*, "From 25 to 30 million healthy, middle-aged Americans are at far higher risk than they and their doctors understand them to be, because we're not taking inflammatory factors into account."[19]

Indeed, some doctors believe that CRP is a more accurate indicator of cardiovascular risk than LDL-C, especially in women.[16] Dr. Sinatra states:

> C-reactive protein (CRP) may be the most predictive for cardiovascular killers such as heart attack, stroke, and vascular disease. Studies have shown that people with elevated CRP run two times the risk of dying from a cardiovascular-related problem compared with those who have high cholesterol levels. Combine a cholesterol burden with a markedly elevated CRP and your risk of heart attack and stroke increases by a factor of nine.[18]

While research continues on defining the actual importance of CRP as an indicator of cardiovascular risk, some experts believe that inflammation, as reflected by CRP, has always been the major factor underlying atherosclerosis. Dr. Uffe Ravnskov and others have written extensively about the holes in the cholesterol theory and that mainstream medicine's obsession with reducing cholesterol levels has always been misguided. Dr. Ravnskov believes that statins work via their antioxidant, anti-inflammatory, and anti-clotting effects. If this were true, it would warrant a less aggressive approach with statins because CRP levels respond to lower statin doses. Thus, Dr. Ravnskov advises, "It may be wiser to search for the lowest effective dose instead of the dose with maximal effect on LDL-cholesterol."[20] The issue of statin dosing is key to using these drugs effectively and safely, and will be discussed in depth in subsequent chapters.

The American Heart Association and the U.S. Centers for Disease Control and Prevention now recommend CRP tests for people at risk for cardiovascular disease. A CRP level below 1 is low risk; 1–3 moderate risk; above 3 high risk. Some doctors are already ordering CRP tests on all patients and prescribing statins drugs to everyone with an elevated level of CRP, yet many experts believe that prescribing drugs is premature. "Before we have tens of millions of Americans placed on statins because of their CRP, we need randomized clinical trials to show they would benefit," Dr. Sidney Smith, professor of medicine at University of North Carolina at Chapel Hill and chief science officer at the American Heart, told *The Wall Street Journal*.[21]

CRP levels are improved by the same factors that improve cardiovascular health: exercise, good diet, maintaining a healthy weight, and not smoking. Women should be aware that hormonal therapy for menopausal symptoms might raise their CRP level considerably.[22] Aspirin appears to be effective for reducing CRP, probably due to its anti-inflammatory effect. But the big push today for treating elevated CRP is with statins. However, before rushing to prescribed drugs for elevated CRP, shouldn't we be asking why CRP levels are elevated in the first place?

One possibility is that our diets are deficient in nutrients needed by humans to maintain a healthy balance between pro-inflammatory and anti-inflammatory systems. The main nutrient for maintaining anti-inflammatory effect is omega-3 oils from fish and whole grains. The western diet is terribly deficient in omega-3 oils. Meanwhile, westerners get huge amounts of omega-6 oils (safflower, sunflower, corn, soy, peanut oils) that have a pro-inflammatory effect. Could it be that we are seeing higher incidences of many types of inflammatory disorders like rheumatoid arthritis, lupus, Crohn's disease, and markers like elevated CRP because our diets are skewed toward pro-inflammatory nutrients?

The proper balance between omega-6 (O6) and omega-3 (O3) oils in the human diet should be 2:1 or even 1:1. In the U.S., it is 17:1. With people eating so many pro-inflammatory oils decade after decade, is it really surprising that we are seeing a tide of inflammatory disorders today? In comparison, in Greece the O6/O3 ratio is 2:1, and the incidence of cardiovascular disease is much lower.[23, 24] (For more on omega-3 oils, see Chapter 9.)

There are other reasons not to prescribe statins to every person with elevated CRP. We are just learning about this indicator and what influences it. For example, a study in the *Journal of the American College of Nutrition* demonstrated that 515 mg/day of vitamin C reduced CRP by 24 percent.[25]

Might vitamin C alone or combined with fish oils or other natural anti-inflammatories reduce CRP as much as statins? It would be much cheaper, safer, and physiologically beneficial to the body. These and many other questions await further study.

OTHER RISK FACTORS

As if it is not already complicated enough, several other factors have now been linked with an increased risk of atherosclerosis, heart attacks and strokes, and premature cardiovascular death.

Triglycerides

Although not a type of cholesterol, triglycerides, like cholesterol, are common fats in the body. Elevated blood levels of triglycerides are directly linked to heart attacks and strokes, and the risk is magnified if you also have a high LDL-C, low HDL-C, or a preponderance of small, dense LDL-C particles. Your fasting triglyceride level should be below 150 mg/dl. A borderline triglyceride level is 150–199; elevated, 200–499; extremely high, over 500 mg/dl.

High carbohydrate diets and alcohol can exacerbate triglyceride problems, so treatment includes moderate carbohydrate intake and alcohol avoidance, as well as weight loss and smoking cessation. Although statins can reduce triglyceride levels, niacin and other drugs are usually used first. Omega-3 oils also reduce triglycerides and might be considered before drug therapies.

Small Particle LDL-Cholesterol

Small particle LDL-cholesterol is a newly recognized risk factor for heart disease. LDL-C particles in the bloodstream come in various sizes. The body can metabolize large particles quickly, but small, dense LDL-C particles can attach to atherosclerotic plaques, increasing plaque size. Indeed, new studies suggest that longevity may be linked more closely to having large LDL-C and HDL-C particles rather than low LDL-C levels. Testing for LDL-C particle size is not routinely done, but it may be useful if you have a family history of heart disease, because the tendency toward small particle LDL-C is usually genetically determined. Small particle LDL-C is worsened by a high carbohydrate/low-fat diet if it raises your triglyceride level. Simple carbs are the main culprit and should be avoided (see Chapter 10). Weight loss and exercise can help reduce small-particle LDL-C levels. Niacin is the most effective pill treatment (see Chapter 8).

Lipoprotein A

Lipoprotein A consists of a molecule of LDL linked with a protein (apoprotein A). An elevated level of lipoprotein A is a major risk factor for coronary artery disease. Some practitioners believe it may be the most important single risk factor in assessing cardiovascular risk. An elevated lipoprotein A is usually genetically determined and found in about 20 percent of the population. Most doctors do not routinely screen for elevated lipoprotein A, but testing for this factor should be considered for at-risk individuals or those with family histories of heart disease or stroke. Recent reports also suggest that lipoprotein A is a major risk factor in older people.[26, 27] Mainstream medical dogma states that diet and weight loss do not affect lipoprotein A levels very much, but some alternative practitioners report significant lipoprotein A reductions with strict elimination diets.[28] Niacin appears to be the only reliable treatment for reducing lipoprotein A levels. Statins are not believed to affect lipoprotein A significantly. However, a recent anecdotal report suggests that statins can actually increase lipoprotein A in some people.[26]

Homocysteine

An elevated homocysteine level is linked not only to coronary artery disease and congestive heart failure, but also to impaired cognitive functioning and Parkinson's and Alzheimer's diseases in the elderly, pregnancy complications, birth defects, increased death rates in diabetics, and possibly cancer. Elevated homocysteine levels may indicate abnormal functioning of the inner lining of blood vessels (the endothelium) and, possibly, an increased tendency for clotting. People with elevated homocysteine levels have a much greater risk of having heart attacks or dying of heart disease than people with normal homocysteine levels. As many as 20 percent of people with heart disease and 30 percent of people with other cardiovascular diseases have high values of homocysteine.

Homocysteine accrues in harmful amounts in people who are unable to metabolize the amino acid methionine. Methionine is abundant in meat, so reducing meat intake lowers homocysteine levels in these people. Dr. Kilmer S. McCully, who discovered the homocysteine-artery disease link in 1969, believes that atherosclerosis is primarily a disease of protein metabolism from the excess protein in western diets.[29] According to McCully, limiting animal protein, caffeine, and alcohol, and performing exercise and stress reduction can reduce homocysteine levels substantially.

Folic acid is very effective in facilitating the metabolism of methionine, thereby reducing homocysteine levels; vitamins B_{12} and B_6 also assist. On the other hand, niacin can raise homocysteine levels in some people, so your homocysteine level should be checked if you take niacin. (For guidelines about healthy homocysteine levels and the use of folic acid, see Chapter 9.)

Fibrinogen

Elevated fibrinogen in the blood is linked to an increased risk of strokes, heart attacks, and cardiovascular death. Fibrinogen is a protein involved in clotting, and it seems to make platelets stick more readily to atherosclerotic plaques or to form clots when these plaques rupture. Elevated fibrinogen levels are more predictive of cardiovascular risk for women than for men. Mainstream doctors and some alternative doctors recommend aspirin (81 mg daily) to reduce platelet clumping and clotting in at-risk patients, because studies have proven that aspirin can reduce their risk of heart attacks and atherosclerotic strokes. Other alternative doctors recommend omega-3 fatty acids (fish oils), arginine, bromelain, vitamin E, garlic, or turmeric or curcumin (a turmeric extract).

HOW MUCH CHOLESTEROL REDUCTION DO YOU REALLY NEED?

Scientists have been studying cholesterol and atherosclerosis for half a century, but we are still learning how complicated it is. And although new technologies are producing a revolution in our understanding of cardiovascular disease, there's no unanimity on whether we are being too aggressive with statins or not aggressive enough. Dr. William C. Roberts, the Editor-in-Chief of the *American Journal of Cardiology,* argues that our cholesterol guidelines are not stringent enough.[2] Atherosclerosis and coronary disease are preventable, Dr. Roberts states. Because relatively little cardiovascular disease is seen in people with total cholesterol levels below 150 and LDL-C levels below 100 mg/dl, Roberts and others argue that these or even lower levels should be everyone's goals.

But many doctors are uncomfortable with placing all patients on powerful drugs like statins, especially at larger and larger doses, for life. Indeed, some experts have begun to question how much extra protection from heart attacks and strokes is really obtained by pushing statins so aggressively.

Sorting this out requires defining who we are talking about. For people with cardiovascular disease or diabetes, the evidence for pushing target levels below 100 mg/dl is strong. For people with a very high risk, such as people with advanced or acute heart disease, the target LDL-C level is now even lower—less than 70 mg/dl. In contrast, for the vast majority in the primary prevention group, especially those with few risk factors, the evidence points in a different direction. For example, consider the study titled "Cholesterol Reductions and Clinical Benefit: Are There Limits to Our Expectations?" Yes, the doctors concluded, there are limits. They wrote: "About two-thirds of the predictable coronary heart disease incidence can be reversed by a 20% to 35% reduction in LDL cholesterol." In fact, it was the first 5–10 percent reduction in LDL-C that provided the greatest benefit. Pushing for extreme reductions in LDL produced diminishing returns. The authors concluded that for people with moderate cholesterol elevations and no cardiac disease, "the mean [LDL-C] reduction does not have to be extreme."[30]

The highly publicized Cholesterol and Recurring Events (CARE) study confirmed these findings. In people with moderate cholesterol elevations, reducing LDL-C to 125 mg/dl significantly reduced coronary problems. But the researchers found "no further decline [in coronary problems] was seen in the LDL range from 125 to 71."[31] Reducing LDL-C to 125 mg/dl was enough.

The extensive West of Scotland Coronary Prevention Study (WOSCOPS) provided similar findings, surprising its researchers. "We hypothesized that larger decreases in LDL-C would be associated with greater benefit. However, no clear, graded relationship was observed." Reducing LDL-C by 24 percent provided "the full benefit of a 45% risk reduction" of coronary heart disease. They added, "further decreases in LDL were not associated with larger reduction in coronary heart disease risk. . . . A fall in the range of 24% [in LDL-C] is sufficient to produce the full benefit in patients."[32]

There is little debate within mainstream medicine that people who have had heart attacks or strokes need intensive treatment. There is little debate that people with very high LDL-C levels coupled with diabetes or multiple risk factors and hypertension are also at greater risk and need treatment. Reaching LDL-C levels of 100 mg/dl or lower makes sense for these people. The debate today swirls around the population with moderate LDL-C elevations, or few risk factors, or no history of cardiovascular disease—in fact, the majority of people with elevated cholesterol. Even in these low-risk or moderate-risk people, some doctors push for LDL-C levels of 100 mg/dl or lower by prescribing strong doses of statins. Others seek more modest goals of LDL-Cs of 130 or 160 mg/dl, as current guidelines recommend. Others believe that no treatment is usually necessary. Dr. Sinatra advises, "If you have been diagnosed with heart disease, multiple risk factors in combination such as diabetes or high overall cholesterol, or have had a bypass, statins may be absolutely appropriate. But it is not smart medicine to prescribe statin drugs simply to lower cholesterol in an otherwise healthy person."[18]

Other experts have challenged the use of statins in low-risk people. In an article in the *American Journal of Cardiology*, Dr. P.M. Moriarty noted that the benefits of therapies are often exaggerated when studies report their results in terms of relative risk reduction.[33] For example, a study may conclude that a statin reduces the risk of some people by 25 percent. But if the overall risk is small in the first place, as in people with moderately high cholesterol levels and few risk factors, then the actual benefit of the statin is quite small. Indeed in an evidence-based analysis funded by the Ministry of Health of British Columbia, Canada, a review of recent studies of statins and primary prevention patients revealed that "statins have not been shown to provide an overall health benefit in primary prevention trials."[34]

In fact, even for some patients with cardiovascular disease, some studies support a more tempered approach. A large meta-analysis of thirty-eight studies involving 83,000 patients examined various treatments for preventing strokes in coronary patients. The results indicated that statins were clearly the most effective therapy, but these benefits applied only to people with very high cholesterol levels, and only a relatively modest reduction of total cholesterol to 230 mg/dl was necessary for the maximum benefit. More rigorous cholesterol reductions, requiring higher statin doses, provided no additional benefit.[35]

Dr. Ted Ganiats, the chairman of the department of family and preventive medicine at the University of California, San Diego, and a member of the National Cholesterol Education Program Coordinating Committee, told me, "We know that lowering LDL-C works wonders at lowering cardiovascular disease risk. It appears, though, that no matter what the LDL-C level is, the greatest reduction in risk occurs with the first 20% drop in LDL-C. Take two people, one with an LDL-C of 130 and one with an LDL-C of 200. When statins reduce their LDL-C 20%, both will get a big drop in their relative cardiovascular risk. Now, if we increase their statin doses and drop their LDL-C another 20% the risk drops further, but not as much."

Why is this the case? Perhaps because the lower statin dose provides both LDL-C lowering plus important anti-inflammatory effects. The higher dose provides only some additional LDL-C lowering effects. This extra albeit smaller amount of benefit may be crucial if you have advanced coronary disease, which is why the experts now recommend reducing LDL-C by

30 percent to 40 percent in high-risk people, but it may not be worth the risk and cost if you are in the low- or moderate-risk groups.

WHAT YOU SHOULD DO

Where does all of this leave you? Fortunately, beyond the cholesterol controversy, there's little debate that factors such as elevated C-reactive protein, homocysteine, fibrinogen, and lipoprotein A levels, low HDL-C levels, as well as obesity, stress, smoking, and physical inactivity are clear risk factors for cardiovascular disease, and they should be rectified. Even the cholesterol skeptics agree with this and support the use of statins, when appropriate, for these other factors.

What if your cholesterol levels are not elevated, but you have a strong family history of cardiovascular disease or death? You should have all of the other risk factors measured. Triglycerides, CRP, homocysteine, and fibrinogen levels can usually be done at the same time you get cholesterol levels measured. Some mainstream laboratories are now offering the VAP analysis, an in-depth analysis of more than a dozen cardiovascular risk factors including those mentioned above as well as lipoprotein A and small particle LDL-C. Most likely, one or more of these levels will be elevated, and you should have it treated.

What should you do if you have elevated cholesterol or LDL-C? My opinion is that, at this point, the weight of scientific evidence supports the effort to lower elevated LDL-C levels. Maybe someday, cholesterol levels will be replaced by more sophisticated measures of cardiovascular risk. Today, the evidence suggests that not only is LDL-C an important risk factor, but that most of the other risk factors become far more dangerous when coupled with an elevated LDL-C. Thus, for now I think it is prudent to achieve your target LDL-C level according to the NCEP guidelines (see pages 24–25).

However, I also believe that many people with elevated cholesterol have nutritional imbalances, not medical disorders. If you have a mild-to-moderate LDL-C elevation, it is better to reduce LDL-C via a heart-healthy diet and to lower overall risk by maintaining a healthy weight, exercising, and not smoking. In an optimal healthcare system, we would start with these interventions first, followed by natural supplements, and then medications if needed. Unfortunately, today we usually take the opposite approach, medicalizing and then medicating without sufficient consideration for more natural, more physiologic alternatives.

Fortunately, there's a lot you can do on your own. A heart attack is often a person's first warning that he or she has cardiovascular disease, so it is important to take preventive measures now. If you are at risk, there's a lot you can do to reduce it. In fact, you can order your own tests and buy supplements that can lower cholesterol or other risk factors, and low-dose statins may soon be available over the counter. But assessing cardiovascular risk can be complicated, so I always recommend working with the guidance of a knowledgeable professional.

If you do need statin therapy, ask your doctor: How much LDL-C lowering do I really need? Listen closely, because some doctors treat everyone aggressively with statins, even if you only need a moderate reduction in LDL-C. Most doctors prescribe the strong initial doses recommended in package inserts and the PDR to all patients whether you are big or small, young or old, healthy or taking eight other drugs. Yet these standard doses are excessive for millions of people. A woman was prescribed 10 mg of Lipitor by her doctor, but she had heard me speak and insisted on starting with 5 mg. She was 79 and weighed 105 pounds. Her LDL-C dropped from 140 to 82 mg/dl, a 41 percent reduction. And by cutting her dose in half, she cut her costs in half, too.

Everyone is not the same. Many people get large LDL-C reductions with tiny statin doses, but many doctors are not aware of this because they have never seen the data. The only way for you or anyone to know how well you might respond to a low-dose statin is to try it. This is the precision-prescribing method. If a low dose does not work, it can easily be increased. The precision-prescribing method is the only one that guarantees that you will get the precise amount of medication you need.

The statin dose is something you should question your doctor about thoroughly. Be sure to ask: What is the lowest statin dose that can accomplish my goal? Your doctor may not know, because drug companies often omit this information from package inserts, the PDR, and the promotional materials given to doctors by drug company sales reps. This is why I have written *What You Must Know About Statin Drugs & Their Natural Alternatives*: to provide sound, evidence-based strategies for you and your doctor when making these decisions. Today, there is so much information, and doctors have so little time, more and more patients are taking the initiative in learning about their disorders and bringing reliable, evidence-based information to their doctors—the kind of quality information that most doctors will heed. By doing this, you can develop a true patient-doctor relationship and obtain the best and safest treatment for yourself and your family—and maybe for your doctor's subsequent patients as well.

3

The Right Statin at the Right Dose

Applying the Precision-Prescribing, Start-Low Go-Slow Method With Statins

It's long been known that for individual subjects the dosage listed on a drug label is not necessarily the right one.[1]

—CARL PECK, DIRECTOR OF THE DRUG DEVELOPMENT CENTER
AT GEORGETOWN UNIVERSITY

Once you have determined how much of an LDL-C reduction you require, it is decision time. But before your doctor selects a drug and dose based on the information in a package insert or in the *Physicians' Desk Reference*, you need to know that those guidelines may not be right for you. I have written extensively on why the doses selected by drug companies are too strong for millions of people.[2-7] This is a widespread problem involving many top-selling drugs, including antidepressants, antihypertensives, anti-inflammatories, antihistamines, anti-anxiety drugs, sleep medications, hormones, gastrointestinal drugs, pain medications—and statins.

THE DEVIL IS IN THE DOSAGE

Most doctors know little about how drug companies actually decide on the doses they recommend. Few doctors know the huge influence of drug companies' marketing divisions on medical decisions like drug doses. A few experts have commented on this problem before. One of them is Dr. Peck, quoted above, who has been writing about the problem since the early 1990s when he was the Director of the Center for Drug Evaluation and Research of the U.S. Food and Drug Administration. Dr. Peck writes: "There are noteworthy examples in drug development of failing to get the dose right when a drug is first marketed."[8]

My colleague, Dr. Andrew Herxheimer, of the renowned Cochrane Centre in Britain, has also been concerned about this problem for many years. He writes:

> Drugs are often introduced at a dose that will be effective in around 90% of the target population, because this helps market penetration. The 25% of patients who are most sensitive to the drug get much more than they need.[9]

With statins, the number is closer to 40 percent.[10] Yet instead of getting better over the years, the problem is getting worse, according to James Cross, former Regulatory Health Project Manager of the FDA's Office of New Drugs. After publishing a study on the problems with standard doses, he stated:

> We've seen a lot of situations where drugs are approved by the FDA and subsequent important information about their optimal dose is not determined until afterward.[1]

Why is this happening? Whenever I speak, someone asks: "Why would drug companies want to overmedicate people?" They don't. So why are the standard statin doses that drug companies recommend and doctors prescribe too strong for so many people? There are many reasons for this. Drug company studies establishing doses are often too small and too brief. The subjects are usually younger and healthier than everyday office patients, and these subjects need and tolerate stronger doses than the average patient. With statins, the initial doses recommended in the PDR are based mainly on studies of people with serious cardiac disease or highly elevated cholesterol levels. Yet the average person with high cholesterol has mild-to-moderate elevations and few risk factors, and therefore does not require such strong doses.

Perhaps the biggest reason is that drug companies like to market drug doses that are strong enough to impress doctors with their effectiveness and to appear superior to competitors' drugs. Powerful doses make better advertising. For years, Lipitor's advertising boasted: "More power to reduce LDL at the 10-mg starting dose than Zocor 10 mg, Pravachol 20 mg, and Mevacor 20 mg in head-to-head trials."[11] Doctors, impressed, soon made Lipitor the top-selling statin. But any statin can provide impressive results with strong doses. The problem is, many people do not need excessively powerful statin doses. More is not necessarily better with medications. Using stronger doses than you need only increases your risks of adverse effects. But strong doses make good advertising copy and improve the bottom line.

Drug companies have also learned that doctors prefer medications that are easy to prescribe, and cookbook, one-size-fits-all dosing guidelines make prescribing quick and easy. So, although doctors are told to use judgment in selecting statin doses, the actual information doctors receive does not support this. Doctors assume that the drug companies and FDA have been diligent in these determinations, and they follow the drug companies' guidelines and prescribe the strong, standard initial doses without a second thought.

Dr. Peck advises otherwise, recommending that doctors "start low and go slow," except of course in medical emergencies.[1] I have been recommending a start-low go-slow approach for decades. Even Robert Ehrlich, the drug industry consultant who designed the highly successful launching of Lipitor, now agrees:

> Why should a 110-pound woman be given the same dose as a 250-pound man? How can the same dose be appropriate for both . . . ? I would ask the drug companies to be more consumer-centric and consider more low dose alternatives. It might work just enough, however, to satisfy the patient and might lead to better patient retention and compliance. Doctors would have more choices in treating their patients. Those doctors who do not want to titrate later can offer the higher doses initially. Those who are willing to start low and monitor patients will have the lower dose available. Sounds like a reasonable alternative.[12]

START LOW, GO SLOW

The practical size of pre-marketing clinical trials means that we cannot learn everything about the safety of a drug before we approve it. Therefore, a degree of uncertainty always exists about the risks of drugs. . . . In many cases drug therapy requires an individualized treatment plan and monitoring.[13]

—U.S. Food and Drug Administration

The start-low go-slow approach is a basic principle of the precision-prescribing model. This model is essential for maximizing the benefits and minimizing the risks with statins because in real life, different people get much different responses from the same dose of the same statin than the drug companies' statistical averages indicate. How can you tell whether you will get a larger or smaller effect than the average? Only by taking a statin yourself. Then you know how your body responds to the drug. Will you get a better-than-average response, a less-than-average response, or side effects? There is no way to know in advance of taking the drug. Medical science acknowledges that despite scores of studies and years of experience with a drug, when an individual takes a new drug for the first time, it is an experiment of its own, and the outcome cannot be foreseen. So the question is, do you want to start with a strong standard dose or a lower, safer, proven-effective statin dose? It is your choice—or at least it should be.

Clinical studies support a start-low go-slow approach because of the wide variability in statin response among people. For example, the standard initial doses of Zocor are 20 and 40 mg. Zocor 20 mg yields an LDL-C reduction of 38 percent. This is what the package insert and PDR tell your doctor. But what is missed is that this is an average reduction derived statistically. The PDR does not tell you about the range of responses seen among actual patients taking Zocor. It does not tell you that in one study, 11 percent of patients obtained 40 percent reductions or greater in LDL-C *with only 2.5 mg of Zocor.*[14] That's ⅛ the standard 20-mg initial dose! Or about another study in which 45 percent of patients were able to reach their LDL-C goal *with just 5 mg of Zocor*—¼ the standard initial dose.[15] Such responses are not unusual, yet they are not usually mentioned in package inserts, the PDR, or the other information doctors receive about statins, or in the drug references used by consumers.

Indeed, low doses of milder statins such as Pravachol and Mevacor have been proven to be surprisingly effective. This information emerged when, a few years ago, the manufacturers of Pravachol and Mevacor sought approval for low-dose, over-the-counter versions of these drugs. The FDA denied their applications not because they were not effective—they were very effective—but because of concerns about people self-medicating with drugs that can cause liver, muscle, or kidney injuries.

In fact, the studies the manufacturers submitted to the FDA were quite impressive. The manufacturer-recommended initial dose of Pravachol is 40 mg/day, yet in the manufacturer's low-dose study using just 10 mg, 83 percent of people with mild-to-moderate cholesterol elevations reached their target LDL-C levels of 130 mg/dl or less.[16] Four studies by Mevacor's manufacturer showed that just 10 mg of the drug, combined with diet counseling, reduced cholesterol successfully in 69 percent to 75 percent of subjects. Indeed, the LDL-C of 17 percent to 26 percent of subjects in the Mevacor studies dropped below 100 mg/dl, the level sought for people with cardiac disease.[17] My point is: Many people get much better LDL-C reductions than the averages indicate, so there is ample scientific basis for a start-low go-slow approach with statins for people who prefer a safety-first approach.

WHO SHOULD USE THE PRECISION-PRESCRIBING METHOD?

The start-low go-slow method is especially suitable if you are in the primary prevention group and have a moderate cholesterol elevation and few risk factors. This group represents the majority of people with elevated cholesterol levels. If you are elderly, small, taking other medications, or have a history of being sensitive to prescription drugs, the start-low go-slow approach is also for you. In fact, the precision-prescribing model is worthwhile for anyone who wants to minimize medication risks. Or, anyone who wants to see how they do with a lower statin dose. In my experience, that is a lot of people—if they are given the option. Usually they are not.

Indeed, even people who need aggressive LDL-C reductions can benefit from the precision-prescribing method. Just because your body requires a large LDL-C reduction does not mean it will tolerate a whopping statin dose from the start. Strong doses are what cause most of the problems with statin drugs. Besides, you might get a much greater LDL-C reduction than expected with a low dose, and starting low avoids overmedication and unnecessary side effects. If a low dose is not strong enough, it can be easily increased. In my experience, people needing strong drug doses still run into fewer problems if they start lower and increase gradually, thereby giving their bodies a chance to adapt to the foreign chemical, rather than starting with a strong dose at once.

Variation with statin drugs can be unpredictable. Many young, large, healthy people also respond to low-dose statins. Because it can be difficult to anticipate your best statin dose or whether you are at risk for statin side effects, a start-low go-slow approach is preferable for any person whose medical condition is not acute and who wants to minimize risk. Starting low and going slow may require an extra visit or telephone contact before arriving at your proper statin dose, but because it prevents side effects that would necessitate extra telephone calls, office visits, and new prescriptions, it usually requires less visits and costs less in the long run. And it helps keep people in treatment, saving them, their families, and their insurers the huge costs of premature cardiovascular diseases that require hospitalizations and surgical interventions.

THE FIRST GOAL OF TREATMENT

The first phase of treatment with statins is a distinct phase that must be conducted thoughtfully. It is no coincidence that half of the people who quit statin therapy do so within three months.[18] This is a sensitive period because it is easy for you to feel overwhelmed. You've been told that you have elevated cholesterol, and that this can cause heart attacks and strokes and reduce your lifespan, that you have to change your diet or lose weight or start exercising or stop smoking, and on top of everything else you have to start taking an expensive drug for the rest of your life. All of these changes are quite an adjustment. The last thing you need is a side effect that causes you discomfort or impairs functioning. When this happens, it all becomes too much of a hassle, and many people get fed up and simply give up. This type of situation can and should be avoided.

The goal of the first phase of treatment is to initiate treatment successfully and comfortably. It is easy to lower cholesterol levels successfully with the potent statins at our disposal, but too often it is forgotten that it must be done comfortably or people will not stick with the treatment program. The first phase of treatment for elevated cholesterol should focus on the factors that you can control and that can reduce your need for medication: diet, exercise, weight, not smoking. If your doctor prescribes a statin, it should be at a dose that will not complicate matters. It should be at a dose that matches the LDL-C reduction you require with consideration for your age, gender, size, and other characteristics. And if it is important to you to avoid potential side effects, treatment should be started with an even lower statin dose to see if you get a response that is better than average.

The strength of the initial dose is particularly important because many side effects occur with the very first doses. Indeed, this is such a common phenomenon in medicine, it has a name: *first-dose reactions*, or *first-dose reactivity*. First-dose reactions are a clear indication that standard doses are too strong for patients. In a few areas of medicine, doctors have adapted by starting with very low doses. This is frequently seen in the treatment of high blood pressure, another cardiovascular disease that is complicated by a very high rate of people quitting treatment, mainly because of side effects. A start-low go-slow approach works well for high blood pressure medication and can work well with statins by avoiding first-dose reactions.

This approach is particularly important for people who are at risk for side effects: elderly or small individuals, people with other medical problems or taking other medications, and the medication-sensitive. An article in *The Journal of the American Medical Association (JAMA)* described the approach perfectly:

> For patients at risk for nonspecific side effects, pharmacotherapy may be undertaken in collaboration with the patient in two discrete phases with distinctly different goals. The goal of the first phase is simply to help the patient tolerate a very low dose of medication; therapy is initiated at doses that may be subtherapeutic, with the objective of allowing the patient to get used to the idea of taking a medication. . . . In the second phase of therapy, the dose is gradually increased into the therapeutic range, acknowledging whenever side effects develop, and coupling this with support and encouragement.[19]

Of course, you can request this approach whether you are at risk or not. A basic desire to avoid side effects is enough reason to request precision-prescribing. These are issues that you and your doctor should discuss together. In Chapter 2, you determined your LDL-C goal. Knowing your LDL-C goal, you can now use Table 3.1 to learn the proper statin doses to accomplish this. For example, if you require a 26 percent reduction in LDL-C, you don't need the strong standard starting 10-mg dose of Lipitor, but only 2.5 or 5 mg. You don't need the standard starting 40-mg dose of Pravachol, but only 10 or 20 mg. Table 3.1 contains the information that you and your doctor require to make informed decisions about statin doses. Remember, these numbers are averages. Your response may be larger or smaller. The only way to tell for sure while minimizing your risk is to start low and go slow.

Starting with a lower dose may be more important to you than to your doctor. Because doctors have seen so much benefit from statins, some have become cavalier or dismissive about side effects. Doctors see so many major problems everyday, they sometimes become inured and forget that garden variety, "minor" side effects are not minor to the person experiencing them. One of the basic principles of the safety-first model is: Minor side effects can have major consequences. When muscle pain, abdominal discomfort, or memory problems cause people to quit statin treatment, the consequences are not minor: premature heart attacks, strokes, and death. These complications are catastrophic, require intensive medical and surgical interventions, and drive healthcare costs way up. Even the drug companies lose when people quit treatment, because billions in sales are lost and their research suffers. Nobody wins when side effects drive people from treatment. So initiating statin therapy successfully without side

TABLE 3.1 LDL-C REDUCTIONS WITH STATIN DRUGS

More is not necessarily better with statins. The initial dose should be based on the amount of LDL-C reduction you need and other risk factors. However, these numbers are averages, and many people get greater responses than those listed here, allowing them to use a lower dose.

Medication/ Dosage	Average LDL-C Reduction	Medication/ Dosage	Average LDL-C Reduction
Crestor (Rosuvastatin)		**Mevacor (Lovastatin)**	
1 mg	34%	10 mg	21%
2.5 mg	41%	20 mg*	27%
5 mg	45%	40 mg	32%
10 mg*	46%–52%	80 mg	40%
20 mg	52%–55%	**Pravachol (Pravastatin)**	
40 mg	55%–63%	10 mg	22%
Lescol (Fluvastatin)		20 mg	32%
20 mg*	22%	40 mg*	34%
40 mg*	25%	80 mg	37%
80 mg	36%	**Zocor (Simvastatin)**	
Lipitor (Atorvastatin)		5 mg	26%
2.5 mg	20%–25%	10 mg	30%
5 mg	27%–29%	20 mg*	38%
10 mg*	39%	40 mg*	41%
20 mg*	43%	80 mg	47%
40 mg*	50%		
80 mg	60%		

* = Manufacturer's recommended initial dose(s).

effects should be the first goal of the entire healthcare apparatus. Unfortunately, today, it is not.

If you want to be sure to get the right statin dose for you, start with Table 3.1. This table is original to this book. You will not find this table or the low-dose information it contains in the PDR or doctors' drug references or consumers' pill books. Most people, including most doctors, have never seen the low-dose data in this table. Few doctors have seen any of the studies proving the effectiveness of low-dose statins. Most doctors think that the information in the PDR is comprehensive, but it is not. I did not realize this either until undertaking my research. This is the reason that you have to investigate your illnesses and medications yourself. Your doctor's decisions are only as good as the information he or she receives. Your doctor cannot prescribe a lower statin dose if he or she doesn't know about it. Good decisions require good information. To apply the precision-prescribing, safety-first model to statin therapy, you need to know which drug and which dose is right for you.

WHICH STATIN IS RIGHT FOR YOU?

The drug companies spend hundreds of millions of dollars on advertising to convince you that their statin is best. They spend much more on advertising, seminars, and sales reps carrying the same message to your doctors. These efforts work, even if the message is questionable. The fact is, the difference between statins is not as great as most people or most doctors think. "The drugs are all relatively similar," Dr. David Waters, chief of Cardiology at San Francisco General Hospital told *The New York Times*. "Whether one sells better than another really depends on marketing."[20]

All statins work the same way, so the key difference usually isn't which drug is used, but which dose is best for you. Yet there are some other important distinctions between statins. When aggressive therapy is needed for people with serious cholesterol or cardiac problems, many doctors prefer Lipitor or Zocor. Higher doses of milder statins such as Pravachol and Mevacor sometimes work, but some secondary prevention patients really do require the high potency of Lipitor or Zocor.

For people with mild-to-moderate cholesterol elevations, Pravachol, Mevacor, and Lescol are preferred. Dr. Stephen Sinatra states, "Pravachol is the statin drug I prescribe most often because it is the weakest of the bunch. We don't need to prescribe large doses of these statins to get results."[21] If Lipitor came in lower doses, it would be a reasonable choice for people with moderate cholesterol elevations. Zocor does come in lower doses, but few doctors are aware of them and their effectiveness. The next chapter provides plenty of information—evidence-based information—on the effectiveness of lower doses of all of the statins.

Crestor, the newest statin, presents a very different picture, a picture that reveals a darker aspect of the medical-pharmaceutical complex and how it works. Crestor is being aggressively marketed as the most potent statin, but few people need such potency with its increased risks of side effects. The last potent statin to hit the market was Baycol, and six years later toxicities and deaths necessitated Baycol's withdrawal in August 2001. History may be repeating itself with Crestor. In March 2004, Public Citizen's Health Research Group petitioned the FDA to ban Crestor because of seven cases of life-threatening acute muscle breakdown known as rhabdomyolysis. In addition, nine patients suffered serious kidney damage or kidney failure while using Crestor. Several of these cases occurred in people taking the standard, drug company-recommended starting dose of 10 mg.[22–24] This is a very powerful dose, yet that is what doctors are prescribing because this is what the manufacturer recommends. As I will explain in greater detail in the next chapter, 10 mg of Crestor is far, far more powerful than needed by most people with elevated cholesterol.

Because of the problems reported with Crestor, some health insurers have already dropped Crestor from their formularies. In November 2004, Dr. David Graham of the FDA told a congressional committee that he considered Crestor unsafe.[28] Public Citizen predicts that Crestor will ultimately be banned.[23] This has not prevented Crestor's manufacturer from mounting one of the most intensive marketing campaigns ever for a new drug. The company launched Crestor with a billion-dollar campaign to convince doctors to prescribe the drug despite the fact that it is not only the most potent statin, but also has the briefest track record and is the least well known.

Appalled by the manufacturer's methods, Dr. Richard Horton, the editor of *Lancet*, wrote, "AstraZeneca's tactics in marketing its cholesterol-lowering drug, rosuvastatin [Crestor], raise disturbing questions about how new drugs enter clinical practice and what measures exist to protect patients from inadequately investigated medicines."[25] This has not stopped the Crestor juggernaut. Soon after its launch, Crestor was garnering 27 percent of all new prescriptions for statin drugs. "Doctors listen to the reps, and they think something new is better than old," Dr. Curt Furberg, professor of public health sciences at Wake Forest University, told *The Wall Street Journal*.[26] With thousands of drug reps delivering their version of the truth about Crestor to doctors' offices and supplying them with boxes of free samples, harried doctors are easily influenced.

I am not surprised by the aggressive marketing of Crestor, nor by the complaisance of doctors prescribing it, nor by the serious reactions associated with the drug. In my previous writings, I revealed the dysfunctional aspects of drug industry marketing and doctors' prescribing, and the great harm that results. What surprises me is how, despite one drug fiasco after another, the system does not change. Crestor may ultimately be banned, but until then, ultra-strong Crestor should be avoided unless you cannot obtain the results you require with any of the other known statins or unless there is a specific need for using Crestor. Usually there is not. So if your doctor writes a prescription or offers you samples of Crestor, decline. And if you are feeling bold, ask your doctor why he or she is suggesting the least-known, most-powerful statin, which already has been linked to multiple toxicities, rather than other better known, apparently safer statins.

In stark contrast to Crestor, there is Mevacor. Mevacor offers two advantages no other statin can match—it is the statin with the longest track record, and it is now available as a generic. Known as lovastatin, generic Mevacor can cost you a great deal less if you check different pharmacies for the best price. I discuss this at much greater length and compare costs of statins and non-drug alternatives in Chapter 11. Let it suffice to say here that if cost is the critical factor in deciding whether you can take a statin, lovastatin may be your answer. It also may be a good choice because Mevacor is a moderately potent statin, and it comes in a wide range of doses.

4

Low-Dose Statins—
The Evidence
The Low-Dose Data
Your Doctor Has Never Seen

What are the lowest effective statin doses and how effective are they? What is the scientific evidence? The standard, drug-company-recommended, initial statin doses may be fine for some people, and others may require even higher doses, but millions of others do fine with lower statin doses. This has been proven in studies that have repeatedly demonstrated a wide range of variation in patients' responses to statin drugs. This variation is now explained by recent information on the pharmacogenetics of statin metabolism, which I will explain in the next chapter.

This same variation has now been demonstrated in doctors' offices. In a large clinical study published in the *American Journal of Medicine*, in which 367 office patients received standard statin doses, 38 percent of the patients obtained improvements in their LDL-C levels that surpassed the average reductions listed in statin package inserts and the PDR.[1] These are the very people who often do well on lower statin doses and who frequently get overmedicated and suffer side effects with standard statin doses.

Unfortunately, the drug industry does not market lower, safer, proven-effective doses of some of the most important statins, and no statin manufacturer provides enough information for doctors or patients about the treatment options with low-dose statins.[2] Instead, because of the cookbook guidelines from drug manufacturers, millions of people get statin doses that are double or quadruple their actual need. Thus, overtreatment is common. Undertreatment is common, too, because of inadequate follow-up to make sure that people are getting satisfactory responses to their statins. The precision-prescribing model avoids both these problems. By starting low and going slow, you can be sure to get the exact amount of statin medication you need.

For reducing C-reactive protein, statin dosing is less clear. Studies are now being done, and recommended doses have not been established. So far, it appears that it does not take as much statin medication to lower CRP as to lower a highly elevated LDL-C level. So for CRP, starting with a lower, safer statin dose makes sense. It may make even more sense to try fish oils, vitamin C, or even low-dose aspirin first.

If you require a statin for elevated cholesterol or CRP, starting with a low-dose statin is wise if you have already encountered statin side effects, or if you are small, older, have a history of medication reactions, or simply want to minimize your risks. Starting with a lower dose is not an extreme idea. The U.S. Food and Drug Administration states that for situations in which side effects are a concern, "the recommended starting dose might best be a low dose exhibiting a clinically important effect in even a fraction of the patient population, with the intent to titrate [adjust] the dose upwards as long as the drug is well tolerated."[3] Side effects with statins are common and drive millions of people from treatment. People are right to be concerned about statin side effects.

What are the lowest effective statin doses and how effective are they? What is the scientific evidence that should make your doctor take notice? It is here, and it should be enough to convince any doctor. Also remember that these LDL-C reductions were achieved in carefully done clinical studies. Some subjects in these studies got even greater LDL-C reductions and some lesser reductions than the statistical averages indicate. Your initial dose should be based on the amount of LDL-C reduction you need and your other risk factors. If you want to see if you can get a better-than-average response, or if you want to minimize the risk of side effects, ask your doctor about starting with an even lower dose. Sometimes a low dose is surprisingly effective, yet if it isn't enough, your doctor can easily increase it according to the precision-prescribing method until you arrive at the precise dose for you. As I will repeat again and again, it ultimately makes little difference whether you require a low or moderate or high dose of a statin: what matters is that you get the right dose for you and nothing more.

LOW-DOSE LIPITOR

From 1997 to 2001, the standard initial dose of Lipitor was 10 mg/day, a dose so powerful that it reduces LDL-C an average of 39 percent.[4] Some people get 45 percent or 50 percent LDL-C reductions with this dose. Remember, most people with high cholesterol have moderate cholesterol elevations and few risk factors, and need only 20 percent to 30 percent LDL-

C reductions. Yet in 2002, even stronger initial doses—20 and 40 mg—were approved. I have already received reports of people who were started on 20 mg or 40 mg of Lipitor, yet only needed 5 mg.

Part of the problem is that although 20 percent to 30 percent of LDL-C reductions can often be achieved with just 5 mg or 2.5 mg of Lipitor, there is not a word about these lower, safer, proven-effective doses in the Lipitor package insert or PDR, and the smallest pill is 10 mg. Thus, most doctors don't know how effective low-dose Lipitor is and instead think that 10 mg is the lowest effective dose, so that's where they start most patients when prescribing Lipitor.

Here are some studies you can show your doctor about low-dose Lipitor.

- *Arteriosclerosis, Thrombosis, and Vascular Biology:*
  In a randomized, placebo-controlled study, 5 mg of Lipitor reduced LDL-C 29 percent and increased HDL-C 8 percent on average; 2.5 mg reduced LDL-C 25 percent and increased HDL-C 5.4 percent.[5]

- *Netherlands Journal of Medicine:*
  In a randomized, cross-over study, 5 mg daily of Lipitor reduced LDL-C 27 percent on average.[6]

- *JAMA:*
  In this double-blind, placebo-controlled, multicenter trial with 56 patients from ages 26–74, 5 mg of Lipitor reduced LDL-C 33 percent.[7]

- *Arteriosclerosis:*
  In this review of early studies involving 231 patients, 5 mg of Lipitor reduced LDL-C 27 percent and triglycerides by 25 percent; 2.5 mg reduced LDL-C 22 percent on average.[8]

- *Clinical Pharmacology and Therapeutics:*
  In a randomized, double-blind study, 2.5 mg of Lipitor reduced LDL-C by 22 percent on average.[9]

TABLE 4.1 AVERAGE DOSE RESPONSE WITH LIPITOR			
LIPITOR (ATORVASTATIN) DOSAGE	AVERAGE LDL-C REDUCTION	LIPITOR (ATORVASTATIN) DOSAGE	AVERAGE LDL-C REDUCTION
2.5 mg	20%–25%	20 mg*	43%
5 mg	27%–29%	40 mg*	50%
10 mg*	39%	80 mg	60%

*Manufacturer's recommended initial doses.

LOW-DOSE ZOCOR

Merck's recommended starting dose for Zocor used to be 5 mg/day and 10 mg/day, but in 1998, perhaps to compete with its powerful new rival, Lipitor, Merck doubled its recommended initial doses of Zocor. The recommended starting doses today are 20 mg and, for people requiring large LDL-C reductions, 40 mg. Doctors usually prescribe the 20 mg dose initially, which reduces LDL-C an average of 38 percent. Yet most people with high cholesterol have moderate cholesterol elevations and few risk factors, and need only 20 percent–30 percent LDL-C reductions.

As demonstrated by the following studies, this can often be accomplished with 5 mg or 10 mg, or sometimes just 2.5 mg of Zocor:

- *Physicians' Desk Reference:*
  Merck itself tells doctors that 10 mg of Zocor reduces LDL-C 30 percent and raises HDL-C 12 percent; 5 mg reduces LDL-C 26 percent and raises HDL-C 10 percent on average.[4]

- *Cardiology:*
  In a double-blind, placebo-baseline study, 45 percent of people taking 5 mg/day of Zocor reached target LDL-C of 130 or less. With 10 mg Zocor, 59 percent reached target LDL-C.[10]

- *Journal of Cardiovascular Pharmacology:*
  In an 8-week, placebo-controlled, multicenter study of 166 subjects, 10 mg of Zocor reduced LDL-C 31–34 percent, 5 mg reduced LDL-C 20–29 percent, and just 2.5 mg reduced LDL-C 19–23 percent. In fact, 11 percent of the people taking 2.5 mg/day of Zocor achieved 40 percent or greater LDL-C reductions.[11]

- *Journal of Family Practice:*
  In this fifty-four-week, multicenter, controlled study involving 344 people with severe LDL-C elevations averaging 210 mg/dl, 41 percent of patients reached their target LDL-C with only 10 mg of Zocor.[12]

TABLE 4.2 AVERAGE DOSE RESPONSE WITH ZOCOR			
ZOCOR (SIMVASTATIN) DOSE	AVERAGE LDL-C REDUCTION	ZOCOR (SIMVASTATIN) DOSE	AVERAGE LDL-C REDUCTION
5 mg	26%	40 mg*	41%
10 mg	30%	80 mg	47%
20 mg*	38%		

*Manufacturer's recommended initial doses.

There are many more studies supporting low-dose Zocor, but if these are not enough to convince your doctor, nothing will.

LOW-DOSE PRAVACHOL

Pravachol's manufacturer now recommends a starting dose of 40 mg/day, which reduces LDL-C an average of 34 percent. This dose may be proper for people with coronary disease or highly elevated cholesterol levels, but it is excessive initially for many people with mild-to-moderate cholesterol elevations and few risk factors. For many years, Pravachol's manufacturer recommended 10 or 20 mg/day as the initial doses, but as newer, stronger statins have been marketed, the standard initial dose of Pravachol, like that of Zocor, has been increased. Yet 20 mg of Pravachol reduces LDL-C 30 percent to 32 percent, which is more than sufficient for most people with moderate cholesterol elevations.[3] Being less potent than the standard starting doses of Lipitor or Zocor, 20 mg of Pravachol is less likely to provoke dose-related adverse effects.

Then again, 10 mg of Pravachol may be all you need, as these studies demonstrate:

- *PREDICT Study:*
  Bristol-Myers Squibb sought Food and Drug Administration approval for the over-the-counter use of Pravachol 10 mg. The application was denied because statins were not deemed safe enough for self-use. Still, the study demonstrated the effectiveness of Pravachol 10 mg, which reduced LDL-C 18 percent–22 percent on average. Some people got 30 percent–35 percent LDL-C reductions. The study concluded that 10 mg of Pravachol "brought 83 percent of the over-the-counter population to their National Cholesterol Education Program-defined LDL-C goals."[13]

- *Cardiology:*
  In a double-blind, placebo-baseline study, 33 percent of people taking 10 mg/day of Pravachol reached target LDL-C of 130 or less.[11]

- *Physicians' Desk Reference:*
  10 mg of Pravachol reduces LDL-C 22 percent, and 20 mg reduces LDL-C 32 percent on average.[4]

- *Clinical Cardiology:*
  In this placebo-controlled, double-blind study, 10 mg Pravachol reduced LDL-C 22.4 percent; 5 mg reduced LDL-C 19.2 percent on average.[14]

Another sign of how differently people can respond to Pravachol: Among healthy people, peak blood levels of Pravachol vary six-fold.[10] This 600 percent variability helps explain why people vary so much in their responses to statins—and why doses need to be tailored for each person individually.

TABLE 4.3 AVERAGE DOSE RESPONSE WITH PRAVACHOL			
PRAVACHOL (PRAVASTATIN) DOSE	AVERAGE LDL-C REDUCTION	PRAVACHOL (PRAVASTATIN) DOSE	AVERAGE LDL-C REDUCTION
10 mg	22%	40 mg*	34%
20 mg	32%	80 mg	37%

*Manufacturer's recommended initial dose.

LOW-DOSE MEVACOR

Introduced in 1987, Mevacor was the first statin. Merck recommends 20 mg as the usual starting dose, but the company recommends 10 mg for people needing LDL-C reductions of less than 20 percent.

However, as the following studies demonstrate, the 10-mg dose can be surprisingly effective for people with higher LDL-Cs:

- *FDA Advisory Committee Hearing:*
  Merck also sought approval for an over-the-counter, 10-mg dose of Mevacor, so it submitted four studies of middle-aged people with moderate cholesterol elevations to the FDA. Just 10 mg of Mevacor and diet counseling allowed 69 percent to 75 percent of the subjects to reach their target LDL-C of below 130—and 17 percent to 26 percent achieved an LDL-C below 100 mg/dl.[15]

- *American Journal of Cardiology:*
  In twenty-eight people with total cholesterol levels of 200–240 mg/dl, 10 mg of Mevacor reduced LDL-C 24 percent on average, bringing twenty-seven people to an LDL-C of 130 mg/dl or lower. The authors stated: "Achievement of desirable values of cholesterol with 10 mg of Mevacor was accompanied by less adverse effects and with significant financial saving."[16]

- *JAMA:*
  10 mg of Mevacor was effective for postmenopausal women with moderate cholesterol elevations.[17]

TABLE 4.4 AVERAGE DOSE RESPONSE WITH MEVACOR			
MEVACOR (LOVASTATIN) DOSE	AVERAGE LDL-C REDUCTION	MEVACOR (LOVASTATIN) DOSE	AVERAGE LDL-C REDUCTION
10 mg	21%	40 mg	32%
20 mg*	27%	80 mg	40%

*Manufacturer's recommended initial dose.

LOW-DOSE LESCOL

Lescol comes in only two sizes and its effects are mild at these doses. Twenty mg of Lescol reduces LDL-C an average of 22 percent; 40 mg reduces LDL-C about 25 percent. These numbers cannot compare with the potency of Lipitor or Zocor, but Lescol's mildness may be an advantage for people with moderate cholesterol elevations and few risk factors.

The following study demonstrates the effectiveness of low-dose Lescol:

- *Journal of Family Practice:*
  In this fifty-four-week, multicenter, controlled study involving 344 people with average LDL-C of 210 mg/dl, 20 mg of Lescol brought 16 percent of subjects to their target LDL-C.[12]

TABLE 4.5 AVERAGE DOSE RESPONSE WITH LESCOL			
LESCOL (FLUVASTATIN) DOSE	AVERAGE LDL-C REDUCTION	LESCOL (FLUVASTATIN) DOSE	AVERAGE LDL-C REDUCTION
20 mg*	22%	80 mg	36%
40 mg*	25%		

*Manufacturer's recommended initial doses.

LOW-DOSE CRESTOR

As discussed in the previous chapter, the introduction of Crestor provides a textbook example of how drug companies capitalize on marketing excessively strong doses. Taking a page from Lipitor's highly successful campaign, Crestor is now being pushed as the strongest statin of all. The manufacturer's recommended initial dose of Crestor is 10 mg/day, which is so strong that its advertising can boast that Crestor is stronger than equivalent doses of any other statin. Yet an even stronger 20 mg starting dose of Crestor is also approved for people requiring large LDL-C reductions.

However, more is not necessarily better with medications, and super-strong Crestor 10 mg is much too strong for most people with moderately elevated LDL-C. Nevertheless, many doctors fall for this advertising ploy and place people on Crestor when lower, milder statins would be not only sufficient, but also safer. Not coincidentally, in my opinion, toxicities have already been reported and Public Citizen has petitioned the FDA to ban Crestor. Remember, most major statin side effects are dose-related.

Crestor 10 mg reduces LDL-C a whopping 46 percent to 52 percent. The manufacturer does recommend a lower 5-mg dose for people requiring "less aggressive LDL-C reductions."[18] In fact, 5 mg of Crestor reduces LDL-C by 42 percent, which is still far more than the initial doses of any other statin, even Lipitor, and far surpasses the needs of most people with elevated LDL-C. Moreover, this 42 percent reduction in LDL-C represents the average LDL-C reduction obtained by study subjects. Many people get even greater reductions with this dosage. In one study, 5 mg of Crestor reduced LDL-C as much as 71 percent in some subjects, yet raised LDL-C 2 percent in others. This is why dosing with statins must be individualized.

Not only is a 71 percent reduction in LDL-C far more than most people need, but some experts believe that reducing LDL-C too much too soon can actually trigger adverse reactions including cognitive, memory, and mood disorders. This is why the precision-prescribing model is so useful, because by starting low and going slow, you can carefully learn whether you are highly sensitive to a statin, instead of provoking side effects from a super-strong standard dose. This might be especially important with Crestor because, per the FDA's analysis, the manufacturer's studies *"provide evidence of adequate efficacy at doses lower than 10 mg, at which safety concerns might be avoided."* Furthermore, the FDA found that "doses below those proposed for marketing have potential clinical utility" and that Crestor's "safe use. . . may require the availability of lower dosage strengths."[19]

What might these lower dose strengths be? Although it is not mentioned in the package insert or Crestor advertising, 2.5 mg of Crestor reduces LDL-C by 40 percent, and just 1 mg reduces LDL-C an average of 34 percent (Table 4.6).[20] These doses are still stronger than effective doses of Pravachol, Mevacor, Zocor, and Lescol, and are certainly strong enough for many people with moderate cholesterol elevations and few risk factors. Indeed, the lead author of this Crestor study stated: "Even at 1 mg/day, rosuvastatin [Crestor] reduced LDL-C by 35%, the same percentage reduction seen with simvastatin [Zocor] 20 and 40 mg" in a landmark study.[21] Yet, rather than starting people with 1 or 2.5 mg of Crestor, most get 10 mg, which is four to ten times more medicine. How many will suffer side effects unnecessarily? Unfortunately, Crestor is not marketed in 1 or 2.5 mg sizes.

Who actually needs Crestor? Hardly anyone. The only people needing Crestor are those very few for whom Lipitor and Zocor are not strong enough. Besides, being the newest statin with the shortest track record, Crestor should be the last choice of any statin drug.

TABLE 4.6 AVERAGE DOSE RESPONSE WITH CRESTOR			
CRESTOR (ROSUVASTATIN) DOSE	AVERAGE LDL-C REDUCTION	CRESTOR (ROSUVASTATIN) DOSE	AVERAGE LDL-C REDUCTION
1 mg	34%	10 mg*	46%–52%
2.5 mg	41%	20 mg*	52% 55%
5 mg	45%	40 mg	55%–63%

*Manufacturer's recommended initial doses.

ALTERNATE LOW-DOSE STRATEGIES

There are other ways to obtain customized treatment with statin drugs. One was suggested by Dr. Iliff of Kansas in a letter to *JAMA:*

> 10 mg of Lipitor is more than enough for 80% of my patients, and often much more than enough. This observation led me several years ago to tinker with a weekly dosage of 20 mg [10 mg twice weekly]. In 25 patients, the average LDL-C level fell 22% from baseline.[22]

These results are not surprising. With Dr. Iliff's method, people were taking an average of 3 mg of Lipitor a day, which provided results equivalent to those shown in clinical studies of Lipitor 2.5 mg.

Even if you require a standard statin dose, there is considerable cost savings in using an every-other-day approach. Statins are long-acting drugs, so they are effective when used every other day. For example, rather than using 10 mg of Lipitor each day, you can use 20 mg every other day with virtually the same results. This was shown in a study published in the *American Heart Journal* in October 2002, in which Lipitor not only reduced LDL-C effectively, but the cost savings with the every-other-day approach was 34 percent.[23]

The point is: there are strategies—such as lower doses, every-other-day dosing, mild vs. strong statins—that allow great flexibility when you and your doctor make decisions about statin therapy. Getting the right drug, dose, and method for each person should be the goal. Most cholesterol problems are not emergencies. There is time to see whether an improved diet can substantially reduce your cholesterol level. There is time to see whether a lower, safer statin dose that will not provoke side effects is enough for you. If a low dose is not sufficient, it can easily be adjusted higher.

Some people do need higher statin doses, yet in my experience, even these people encounter fewer side effects if they start low first. It can be harsh on some people's systems to start with 40 mg of Lipitor or Zocor. Starting lower allows their systems to adjust more gradually, successfully. On the other hand, some people start statins at high doses without difficulty. Many of these differences in statin response reflect the differences in people's genetics, which controls the cytochrome P450 enzymes and other systems for metabolizing these drugs. This is explained in greater depth in the next chapter. For now, it suffices to say that we know that different people metabolize statins at very different rates, so the science supporting the use of the precision-prescribing method is strong.

Thus, the key to using statins safely and effectively is for you and your doctor to consider the many options and choose according to your history of medication use and reactions, clinical condition, and preference. If you are concerned about minimizing the risks with statin drugs, you and your doctor can do so by starting low. A start-low go-slow approach assures you of finding your best dose, that is, the least amount of medication that you require with the least risk.

ANOTHER LOW-DOSE APPROACH: COMBINATION THERAPY

To prevent or reduce side effects with statins, many doctors prescribe a lower-dose statin with a low dose of another type of cholesterol-lowering agent. In a study published in the *New England Journal of Medicine,* people with coronary heart disease received 10 mg of Zocor (a few received 20 mg) and extended-release niacin. With this low-dose combination, LDL-C levels dropped 42 percent and HDL-C rose an average of 26 percent. Over three years, these patients saw a 60 percent to 90 percent reduction in their risk of major coronary effects.[24] The manufacturer of Zocor and Mevacor now markets a drug, Advicor, that contains 20 mg of Mevacor with a range of doses of extended-acting niacin. Combining statins and niacin can have complications, so do not add niacin or a niacin derivative to your statin therapy without your doctor's guidance.

In another study, people received 20 mg of Lescol plus 8 mg of cholestyramine (a resin that blocks cholesterol absorption from the intestine). On average, their LDL-C levels fell 31 percent.[25] Today, cholestyramine has been supplanted by Welchol and Zetia, which also block cholesterol absorption and cause fewer apparent side effects. Doctors frequently combine one of these with a lower-dose statin.

I asked a respected internist about this strategy. He replied:

A lot of my patients get dull, aching muscles with statins. Their CPK levels [creatinine phosphokinase, a marker for muscle injury] are normal, but we know that statins can affect muscles and joints anyway. So I have them take Zetia to reduce dietary cholesterol absorption, and I combine it with a low-dose statin to reduce metabolic cholesterol. This works fine. Combining two drugs at low-dose is standard for treating hypertension, and it works well for treating hypercholesterolemia.

Zetia alone reduces LDL-C 18 percent to 24 percent. Many people who have encountered repeated difficulties with statins seem to do fine with Zetia. Zetia does not increase HDL-C or decrease triglycerides, but combining it with a lower-dose statin to achieve a greater reduction of LDL-C makes sense. Vytorin does just that. This new drug contains 10 mg of Zetia and a range of doses of Zocor from 10 to 80 mg. So far, reported side effects seem to be few and mild, but a recent analysis of FDA data by Public Citizen revealed serious adverse effects with Zetia involving muscle, liver, and other organ systems. Public Citizen advises against the use of Zetia, especially in combination with a statin.[36]

Plant sterols and stanols, which are non-drug nutriceuticals (see Chapter 8), also block cholesterol absorption and could be used with low-dose statins. Plant sterols/stanols are less expensive than Zetia and Welchol. Other combinations might include statins with soy or garlic, which have modest cholesterol-lowering effects.

WHEN AGGRESSIVE CHOLESTEROL-LOWERING IS NEEDED

Just as there are people who are very sensitive to statins and need low doses, there are others who are not sensitive and require higher doses. Higher doses are also often needed for people with extremely high cholesterol levels, cardiovascular disease, or multiple risk factors. Some of this variation is due to genetic differences in how people respond to statins, but some of this variation is because people do not adhere to cholesterol-lowering diets, so they do not get as good a response with statins as the averages suggest. Indeed, some people use statins as an excuse for eating more junk rather than using statins as they are meant: as adjuncts to a healthy diet, moderate exercise, and a lifestyle that minimizes cardiovascular risk. The fact is, adhering to these healthful lifestyle strategies is more important than taking a statin.

Even if you need aggressive statin therapy, this does not mean treatment must always be *started* aggressively. Although some people do fine when started on strong statin doses such as 20 or 40 mg of Lipitor or Zocor, others do not, and starting with such strong doses definitely increases side-effect risks. Starting low and increasing gradually minimizes these risks.

The choice of an initial dose should be based not only on your LDL-C level and other risk factors, but also on your age, size, history of medication tolerance or sensitivity, and whether you are taking other medications. It should also be based on how ready you are to take prescription drugs for the rest of your life and how important it is for you to avoid side effects. If you are concerned about avoiding short-term and long-term side effects, you will prefer the precision-prescribing method, which will allow you to reach your best statin dose in a stepwise manner. It is not unusual for people who suffer reactions when initially prescribed strong statin doses to do much better when started again at lower doses, which are then gradually increased. This allows people's systems the opportunity to adjust to the drug. If you remember how strongly your first drink of alcohol or coffee affected you, it is easy to understand that starting any new chemical, including statins, can sometimes be a shock to the system. The point of the precision-prescribing method is to avoid this while allowing you to ultimately reach your treatment goals safely.

INCREASING STATIN DOSES SAFELY

According to the drug companies, statin doses should be increased 100 percent at a time, so that's what doctors do. For example, doctors routinely increase statin doses from 20 to 40 mg. But for people who are near but not quite at their target LDL-C with 20 mg of a statin, a better alternative might be to try 30 mg next. This can be accomplished with 1½ 20-mg pills or a combination of 10 and 20 mg pills. Another method is to take 20 mg one day, 40 mg the next. The same model can be used for going from 10 to 15 instead of 20 mg, or going from 40 to 60 instead of directly to 80 mg. These saved milligrams can add up when taking a statin year after year and can lower your risks of long-term complications.

IF YOU ARE ALREADY TAKING A STATIN

If you are already taking a statin and not having any problems, that's good. That's the goal. Still, because of the possibility of long-term risks, ask your doctor if you might get by with a lower maintenance dose. Sometimes, especially if you have made improvements in diet and exercise, the dose can be reduced. If a lower maintenance dose does not provide enough cholesterol or C-reactive protein reduction, return to your regular dose.

If you are already taking a statin and having side effects, ask your doctor about reducing the dose or switching to a milder statin. If problems persist, you and your doctor might consider one of the non-drug alternatives described in Chapter 8. If you are taking a statin but do not like the idea of needing a prescription drug, there are many non-drug alternatives that work. Non-drug alternatives are reasonable choices for people with mildto-moderate cholesterol or CRP elevations, no cardiovascular disease, and few risk factors. However, for people with severe cholesterol or CRP elevations, or those with histories of major cardiovascular disease, I recommend statins first because they are proven to reduce cardiovascular morbidity and mortality. Whether you use a statin or a non-drug alternative, cardiac health also depends on adequate amounts of nutrients like folic acid, magnesium, and omega-3 oils, which I discuss in Chapter 9, and first and foremost a healthy lifestyle.

LONG-TERM SIDE EFFECTS OF STATINS

There are no guarantees with any drug. Just because a drug is safe for most people does not mean it will be safe for you. And although you may take a drug for years, problems can still develop unexpectedly. Millions of people will take statins for twenty to fifty years. Lipitor, the top-selling statin, has been on the market for eight years. Mevacor, the oldest statin, has been available for eighteen years. So people taking statins today are serving as our test group for long-term risks with these drugs.

So far, statins have proven to be pretty safe overall, but problems have arisen. Baycol, the sixth statin, was withdrawn in 2001 after dozens of people died from acute muscle breakdown. In 2001, a report from France linked Lipitor and Zocor with tendon problems.[26] In 2002, Merck announced a risk of severe, potentially fatal reactions when Zocor is used with the heart drug Cordarone.[27] All of these problems were discovered after the fact—in other words, discovered when patients suffered these reactions with statins.

Discoveries of new problems with statins are almost certain. "Discovery of new dangers of drugs after marketing is common," warned an article in *JAMA*. "Overall, 51 percent of approved drugs have serious adverse effects not detected prior to approval."[28] One of the authors of this study, Dr. Thomas J. Moore, stated in another article, "Our society settles for short-term studies about drugs taken for long-term effects. No system is in place to ensure that drugs intended for long-term treatment ever receive long-term testing."[29] This is why extra caution should be used with statins (and any other drugs) that are taken long-term.

In fact, one long-term problem has already been identified with statins: peripheral nerve injuries. In 2002, a study reported that "people who had taken statins were 4 to 14 times more likely to develop polyneuropathy."[30] Peripheral neuropathies are nerve injuries that produce tingling, numbness, pain, or weakness in the limbs. This reaction occurs in 1 in 2,000 users of statin drugs per year. With about 40 million Americans projected to take statins, that's 20,000 cases of peripheral neuropathies each year. These numbers may be underestimates. I spoke to one woman who developed a neuropathy on a statin. Although her neuropathy caused substantial pain for several months and was clearly related to taking a statin, her doctors denied such reactions were possible. So it is very likely that many of these cases are misdiagnosed and never reported to the FDA.

Most peripheral neuropathies are mild and disappear over a few days or weeks, but some neuropathies are severe with very unpleasant nerve pain and/or severe muscle weakness that can be permanent.[31] One doctor wrote to me about developing a painful neuropathy while taking 40 mg of Lipitor. After stopping the drug, it took months for his pain to abate. The doctor added that his reaction was not an isolated event: five of his patients had also developed neuropathies on statins. A key, yet usually unrecognized, factor in the development of neuropathies with statins is that the risk is cumulative: the higher the dose, the greater the risk. This is another reason why using the lowest statin dose you need is the only safe way to go.

Indeed, some experts wonder whether the inhibition of cholesterol synthesis by statins may cause other long-term problems. The respected *Medical Letter On Drugs and Therapeutics* raised this concern: "Cholesterol is a component of all human cell membranes; the long-term consequences of interfering with its synthesis and the synthesis of related compounds are unknown."[32]

By inhibiting cholesterol synthesis in the liver, statins also inhibit the production of coenzyme Q_{10}, which is involved in energy production in cells, especially heart cells. This, some doctors warn, can lead to heart failure. Dr. Julian Whitaker warns, "CoQ_{10} deficiencies and heart failure go hand in hand. We are seeing heart failure like never before, and I believe that the CoQ_{10} deficiencies caused by our increasing reliance on statin drugs are largely responsible for this epidemic."[33] Dr. Sinatra, one of the first advocates of coenzyme Q_{10}, adds:

> Statins deplete coenzyme Q_{10} (CoQ_{10}), one of your body's most important defenses against heart disease, cancer and premature aging. Lack of CoQ_{10} can lead to serious heart and skeletal muscle damage. That's why muscle dysfunction is often associated with these drugs. If you're on a statin drug, be sure to take 100–200 mg of standard CoQ_{10} or 30–60 mg of softgel CoQ_{10}.[34]

Unfortunately, relatively few mainstream doctors know about this problem or recommend CoQ_{10} when prescribing statins. In June 2002, attorneys for Dr. Julian Whitaker petitioned the FDA to add a warning to statin drugs advising doctors to prescribe coenzyme Q_{10} to patients on statins. The petition stated: "All prescribing physicians and pharmacists need to be informed that statin drugs produce a depletion in CoQ_{10}, which increases the risk of myopathies and which in settings of preexisting CoQ_{10} deficiency, such as congestive heart failure and aging, may worsen markedly myocardial function."[35] Statins' impact on CoQ_{10} is another dose-related effect, so lower statin doses cause less CoQ_{10} depletion.

Will other serious long-term problems emerge with statins? No one knows. Doctors do not like talking about this issue and rarely warn patients of how little we know about the long-term risks of medications. How do you minimize the risks? By making sure that you are using the right statin at the right dose for you and nothing more.

5

Why Do People Respond So Differently to Statin Drugs?
Precision Prescribing and the New Science of Pharmacogenetics

Genetic factors are the major determinants of the normal variability of drug effects and are responsible for a number of striking differences in pharmacological activity.[1]

—GOODMAN AND GILMAN'S PHARMACOLOGIC BASIS OF THERAPUTICS

PHARMACOGENETICS AND POOR METABOLIZERS

There are many reasons why people respond so differently to medications. I have already mentioned age, size, and gender. Differing states of health, different medical disorders, and the use of other medications also enter into the equation. Moreover, differences in drug absorption, cell and tissue sensitivities to drug effects, and kidney function add to the variability among people.

Pharmacogenetics, the new science of how our genes influence drug response, is now revealing the most important factor of all: wide differences in the enzymes that people possess for metabolizing and eliminating drugs. Humans possess multiple families of drug-metabolizing enzymes. These enzymes are located mainly in the liver and to a lesser extent in the wall of the small intestine. The efficiency of each enzyme is genetically determined. Beginning in the 1960s, research in pharmacogenetics has shown that wide variations in these genes underlie much of the individual differences in drug response.

Pharmacogenetics has great potential for refining our methods of medication treatment. An article in *The New England Journal of Medicine* put it best:

The promise of pharmacogenetics, the study of the role of inheritance in the individual variation in drug response, lies in its potential to identify the right drug and dose for each patient.[2]

In other words, precision prescribing. Pharmacogenetics allows us to identify people who are at higher risk with specific drugs. If one of your drug-metabolizing enzymes is inefficient or inactive, your ability to inactivate drugs metabolized by this enzyme will be slowed. People with slow acting variants (alleles) of these metabolic enzymes are known as *poor metabolizers (PM)* or slow metabolizers. Because these people metabolize some drugs slowly, they develop higher and longer-lasting blood levels that can build up and, therefore, often get side effects with standard drug doses. As a medical journal article explained, poor metabolizers *"will achieve excessive plasma concentrations at common dosage schedules, and may thus develop disturbing and even dangerous side effects."*[3] (Emphasis added)

This is why a precision-prescribing, start-low go-slow approach is essential. Although this problem is well understood among experts in pharmacogenetics, it is not well known among practicing doctors, so poor metabolizers frequently have great difficulty getting proper treatment. This is what a 29-year-old, medication-sensitive woman encountered when seeking treatment for depression. Her family doctor recognized that she was a poor metabolizer, but this information did not help her with the specialists.

Over the years she had considerable difficulties in explaining to prescribing physicians that she was a slow metabolizer of antidepressants and its implications for drug dosage. After many problems with side effects on various antidepressants, she decided to drop all drug therapy. . . .[3]

This case was published in 1984. Despite great progress in pharmacogenetics since then, the problem for everyday patients remains the same. This should soon change. Tests are already available that, via a blood sample, can analyze your DNA and identify your pattern of metabolizing enzymes. The accuracy of these tests has not been firmly established, but the potential is unmistakable. This potential was defined in a recent article in *JAMA:*

Pharmacogenetics may be one of the most immediate clinical applications of the Human Genome Project. Some adverse drug reactions caused by genetic variation—previously considered non-preventable—may now be preventable.[4]

THE CYTOCHROME P450 ENZYME SYSTEM

People possess several large groups of metabolizing enzymes. The largest group of drug-metabolizing enzymes is the cytochrome P450 system, which accounts for the vast majority of drug metabolism. Although humans possess more than thirty different cytochrome P450 enzymes, six are responsible for most drug-metabolizing functions. Among these is cytochrome 2D6 (CYP2D6), which metabolizes about 25 percent of all prescription drugs. Pharmacogenetics has identified sixteen different variants of CYP2D6, all with different drug-metabolizing efficiency (see page 67). Many people have an intermediate variant of CYP2D6; these people are called *intermediate metabolizers* (*IM*) and usually do well with standard drug doses or, sometimes, lower doses.

Some people have variants of CYP2D6 that are more efficient than the norm. These people are called fast or *extensive metabolizers* (*EM*): they metabolize drugs very quickly and often require standard or stronger drug doses. A small number of people have an ultrafast, highly efficient CYP2D6 variant; such people are *ultrafast metabolizers* (*UM*) and often require very strong drug doses. Other ultrafast metabolizers have a duplicate set of genes and have duplicate sets of CYP2D6 enzymes.

At the other extreme are the poor metabolizers who have an inefficient CYP2D6 variant or no CYP2D6 enzymes at all. These are the people who tolerate only very low medication doses and who react adversely, sometimes dangerously, to standard doses.

Another cytochrome enzyme responsible for metabolizing many drugs is cytochrome 2C9. Approximately 10 percent of the population have inefficient variants or are lacking CYP2C9 altogether. These people are poor metabolizers of the many drugs processed through this enzyme (see page 66).

Such variations in people's cytochrome P450 systems are not the exceptions, but the rule. Pharmacokinetic testing of large numbers of people reveals a spectrum of profiles, with most people having a combination of cytochrome P450 enzymes that include fast, intermediate, and poor metabolizing variants. People whose enzymes are all intermediate are rare. As one expert, writing in *JAMA*, explains:

> There appear to be remarkable differences among patients in the catalytic activity of enzymes termed [cytochrome] P450. It is increasingly evident that this heterogeneity accounts, at least in part, for the differences among patients in response to many medications.[4]

Some Drugs Metabolized By Cytochrome P450 Enzymes

The use of two or more medications metabolized by the same cytochrome P450 enzyme system may lead to inhibition in the metabolism of one or more drugs. Whenever you receive a new medication, ask your doctor and pharmacist whether it might affect the metabolism of other drugs you are taking.

Cytochrome 1A2

Caffeine
Coumadin (warfarin)
Theophylline
Tylenol (acetaminophen)
Zoloft (sertraline)

Cytochrome 2C9

Lescol (fluvastatin)
Cozaar (losartan)
Coumadin (warfarin)
Dilantin (phenytoin)
Motrin (ibuprofen)
Naprosyn, Aleve (naproxen)
Orinase (tolbutamide)
Voltaren (diclofenac)

Cytochrome 2C19

Mesantoin (mephenytoin)
Prevacid (lansoprazole)
Prilosec (omeprazole)
Valium (diazepam)

Cytochrome 2D6

Codeine
Dextromethorphan
Effexor (venlafaxine)
Haldol (haloperidol)
Inderal (propranolol)
Lopressor (metoprolol)
Paxil (paroxetine)
Prozac (fluoxetine)
Risperdal (risperidone)

Cytochrome 2E1

Alcohol
Isoniazid

Cytochrome 3A4

Lipitor (atorvastatin)
Mevacor (lovastatin)
Zocor (simvastatin)
Biaxin (clarithromycin)
Calan, Verelan (verapamil)
Cardura, Dilacor (diltiazem)
Cyclosporine
Erythromycin
Lidocaine
Nizoral (ketoconazole)
Paxil (paroxetine)
Plendil (felodipine)
Prilosec (omeprazole)
Procardia (nifedipine)
Progesterone
Protease inhibitors (rifonavir, saquinavir)
Prozac (fluoxetine)
Quinidine
Sporonox (itraconazole)
Tagamet (cimetidine)
Tegretol (carbamazepine)
Testosterone
Viagra (sildenafil)
Xanax (alprazolam)
Zoloft (sertraline)

INDIVIDUAL VARIATION WITH STATIN DRUGS

Among statin drugs, Lipitor, Mevacor, and Zocor are metabolized by P450 cytochrome 3A4. Research on CYP3A4 has not yet revealed a clear pattern about individual genetic variation, but it is known that the actual functioning of this enzyme can vary greatly from person to person. Moreover, many drugs can directly inhibit the activity of CYP3A4. These include the antibiotics erythromycin and Biaxin (clarithromycin), antifungals Nizoral (itraconazole) and Sporonox (ketoconazole), birth control pills, protease inhibitors for HIV and AIDS, Tagamet (cimetidine), and the immunosuppressant cyclosporine. Inhibition of CYP3A4 by drugs and other factors can cause marked elevations in plasma levels of Lipitor, Mevacor, and Zocor, increasing the risk of side effects. Also, large quantities of grapefruit juice (a quart or more) can inhibit CYP3A4 and raise these statin drug levels substantially. With drugs that cause direct inhibition with CYP3A4, lower doses of Lipitor, Mevacor, and Zocor should be used until the actual effect is known.

Many other drugs are also metabolized by CYP3A4 (see page 66). Although these drugs are not direct inhibitors of CYP3A4, when taken with Lipitor, Mevacor, or Zocor, these drugs may compete for the same metabolizing CYP3A4 enzymes, thereby slowing drug metabolism and raising blood levels of either drug or both. This is called *competitive inhibition*. On the other hand, there are a few drugs, such as Tegretol and Dilantin, that actually hasten the activity of the CYP3A4 enzyme. These drugs could hasten the metabolism of Lipitor, Mevacor, or Zocor, lowering their blood levels and reducing their effects. This would require a higher statin dose.

Lescol is metabolized primarily by cytochrome 2C9. Through competitive inhibition, Lescol plasma levels may rise significantly when taken with the anti-inflammatory Voltaren (diclofenac), the diabetes drug glyburide, and stomach acid suppressors Zantac, Tagamet, and Prilosec, or other drugs listed under CYP2C9 on page 66. On the other hand, Lescol can inhibit the metabolism of other 2C9-metabolized drugs.[5] If you are using any of these medications, Lescol doses should be chosen accordingly.

POOR METABOLIZERS: CAUTIOUS DOSING WITH STATIN DRUGS

If you are a poor metabolizer of CYP2D6, you should start with a very low dose of Lipitor, Mevacor, or Zocor. If you are a poor metabolizer of CYP2C9, low doses of Lescol are recommended. Better yet, you and your doctor should select a statin that you can metabolize normally or quickly. Or consider Pravachol, which has multiple excretion pathways and is not as affected by inefficient cytochrome P450 enzymes, so drug interactions and competitive inhibition are less likely. Yet people can vary widely in their responses to Pravachol, too.

In fact, in a recent study in *JAMA* of genes involved in cholesterol synthesis, absorption, transport, and statin metabolism, the results revealed that genetic factors caused 7 percent of users of 40 mg/day of Pravachol to get a 22 percent smaller drop in total cholesterol and 19 percent smaller drop in LDL-C than other study subjects.[6] This study was the first involving statins to show that pharmacogenetics can also be used to determine who might obtain better results with one statin versus another. As *The Wall Street Journal* explained it: "In a finding with potentially significant implications for the millions of people taking cholesterol-lowering statins, researchers have discovered that patients with a certain genetic makeup get less benefit from a commonly prescribed drug [Pravachol]."[7] The researchers are currently undertaking a similar, possibly more revealing study with Lipitor.

This is the beauty of pharmacogenetics: It not only can tell us whether you are a fast or slow metabolizer who may require higher or lower doses, but it can also guide you and your doctor toward a drug that might work better with less risk based on your own genetics. A big gap in the system has always been that clinical studies provide a lot of information about large groups and general approaches, but little information about how a specific drug will affect a specific person. This is why, when it comes to selecting the right statin at the right dose for an individual, effectiveness and safety can never be assured—which explains why side effects drive so many people from treatment. Pharmacogenetics will allow us to adapt our broad, general knowledge of drugs to the specific requirements of each person. Medication therapy will become more specific and more accurate—as well as more safe and effective than ever possible before.

ARE YOU SENSITIVE TO MEDICATIONS? GENERAL MEDICATION SENSITIVITIES

For most people, it's not unusual to be sensitive to the effects of one medication or another. Many people get side effects with a few medications, but handle most medications without difficulty. Other people, however, get side effects with drug after drug. They have what I call a *general medication sensitivity*. People with general medication sensitivities encounter problems with many different drugs, and they have long histories of one adverse reaction after another.

I estimate that people with general medication sensitivities comprise about 5 percent to 10 percent of the population, that is, 14 to 28 million Americans. Some doctors dismiss such patients, but other doctors readily acknowledge having patients who display general medication sensitivities.

What Type of Metabolizer Are You?

Variations in people's cytochrome P450 systems aren't the exception, but the rule. Most people have a combination of intermediate, efficient, and poor metabolizing CYP450 enzymes. Very few people have a full array of "normal," intermediate functioning CYP450 enzymes.

Intermediate Metabolizers (IM)	An intermediate metabolizer of a cytochrome P450 enzyme displays average patterns of drug metabolism. These people usually develop plasma levels within expected ranges and do well on standard doses of drugs metabolized by this enzyme.
Extensive Metabolizers (EM)	Extensive metabolizers of a CYP450 enzyme display increased efficiency in metabolizing drugs with this enzyme. These people usually display below average plasma levels, and they may require standard or somewhat higher doses of drugs metabolized by this specific enzyme.
Ultrafast Metabolizers (UM)	A small number of people have ultrafast variants of one CYP450 enzyme or another. Such people usually have a duplicate set of the specific gene and enzyme. Drugs affected by this enzyme are metabolized very quickly, so plasma levels are low. People usually require high doses of drugs metabolized by ultrafast CYP450 enzymes.
Poor Metabolizers (PM)	Poor metabolizers possess an inefficient CYP450 enzyme, or the enzyme is absent altogether. These people develop very high plasma levels with standard doses of drugs metabolized by the specific enzyme. Poor metabolizers require very low drug doses and often develop major reactions when standard doses are prescribed to them.

Pharmacogenetics now confirms that some people are poor metabolizers of many classes of drugs. Other medication-sensitive people may have normal metabolizing enzymes, but may have increased tissue sensitivity to the effects of drugs. There are many variables, and we still don't know enough to explain it entirely. The important thing is to use all of our tools—a good medication history, pharmacogenetics, close observation during treatment—to identify these people and to individualize treatment by starting low and going slow. Otherwise, with standard doses, side effects are inevitable, and these people suffer unnecessarily, quit treatment, and then suffer the consequences of untreated diseases. But who can blame them for stopping treatment? Some people with general medication sensitivities encounter so many side effects, they become almost phobic about taking medications and avoid treatment even when it is medically imperative.

Getting your doctor to recognize that you are medication-sensitive or a poor metabolizer can be difficult. Most doctors still are not adequately informed about pharmacogenetics. As *Melmon and Morrelli's Clinical Pharmacology*, a leading pharmacology reference, warned:

> many physicians are not aware of this [genetic] source of variation and are reluctant to accept that, for certain drugs, genetic factors are important and should be incorporated in their dosage considerations. Unawareness of these common variabilities will continue to result in . . . overtreatment. A substantial number of patients will be affected.[8]

That's just part of the problem. Many doctors, unfortunately, are never taught how to assess side effects properly. They never learned anything about people with general medication sensitivities. And most doctors have never seen the data showing that lower doses work, so they prescribe standard doses to everyone, including poor metabolizers and people with obvious medication sensitivities, thinking they are doing the right thing.

Many doctors are not even trained to take a thorough medication history, but you can furnish this information with the Medical Sensitivity Questionnaire on page 71. By listing the medications you have taken and the side effects you have encountered, this history will provide a picture of your drug sensitivity. For example, if coffee or decongestants make you edgy, so might drugs like Prozac, Paxil, Zoloft, Wellbutrin, Zyban, Claritin-D, Allegra-D, over-the-counter decongestants, and other drugs that can cause anxiety.

Family histories may also indicate a poor metabolizing genetic pattern. As a specialist in women's medicine told me, "If their mothers are sensitive

Medication Sensitivity Questionnaire

Intake forms at doctors' offices usually do not ask about medication side effects (exception: allergies)—yet this is important information. To assist your doctor in discussing this issue, enlarge and copy this table at a copy store, fill it out, and bring it to your next appointment. Be sure to have a copy placed on your chart.

1. Are you sensitive to any prescription or non-prescription drugs? If yes, please list and describe:

2. How are you affected by alcohol? Check one and describe:
   ____ Easily affected   ____ Moderately affected   ____ Not affected

3. Do some drugs make you tired or sleepy? If so, please list and describe:
   Cold or allergy remedies or antihistamines (such as Benadryl, Claritin, Contac, Tavist, Zyrtec, etc.):
   Benzodiazepines (tranquilizers or anticonvulsants, such as Ativan, Klonopin, Valium, Xanax):
   Others (such as motion sickness remedies Dramamine or Bonine, or anti-nausea agents Phenergan or Compuzine).

4. Do some drugs give you energy, or cause anxiety or insomnia? If so, please list and describe:
   Coffee, tea, chocolate, or other caffeine-containing substances:
   Appetite suppressants (prescription or nonprescription):
   Cold or allergy remedies or decongestants (such as Sudafed):
   Others:

5. Have you ever had a reaction to epinephrine (adrenaline chloride, often injected by dentists with pain-numbing medication)? Typical reactions include palpitations, sweating, anxiety, and headaches.

6. Have you had any side effects from any other prescription or nonprescription drugs (such as impaired memory or coordination, blurred vision, headaches, indigestion, diarrhea, constipation, dizziness, palpitations, rashes, swelling, ringing in the ears, other reactions)? If so, please list the drugs and side effects:

7. Overall, how would you describe yourself with regard to medications?
   ____ Very sensitive
   ____ Not particularly sensitive to medications
   ____ Very tolerant, usually require high doses

Adapted from: Cohen, J.S. "Ways To Minimize Adverse Drug Reactions: Individualized Doses and Common Sense Are Key." *Postgraduate Medicine*, Sept. 1999;106:163–72.

to a drug, many of my female patients are sensitive, too." Copy or enlarge and fill out the questionnaire and give one to each of your doctors. Your history of medication reactions then becomes a permanent part of your chart, which you can ask your doctor to consider whenever making decisions about drugs and doses.

Over the years, your medication-sensitivity profile may change. Many people become more sensitive to medications as they age. One pharmacist told me, "Many people over 65 are sensitive to medications. By 75 or 80, they're all medication-sensitive." To allay the fears of some medication-sensitive people, treatment should start with an extremely low dose and increase very gradually, if necessary. This method allows you and your doctor to differentiate a possible adverse drug reaction from your own anxiety.

How low can you start a medication? There is virtually no limit. Consider an example from the *United States Pharmacopoeia* of a woman with Mediterranean fever, a rare, potentially lethal autoimmune condition that responded only to an old-time drug, colchicine. At standard doses, colchicine causes abdominal pain or diarrhea in 80 percent of patients. The woman could not tolerate colchicine, but her doctor understood that these side effects were dose-related, so he employed an extreme low-dose approach. He had a pharmacist make a solution of colchicine and gave the woman $1/1000$ of the standard dose. This minuscule amount had no effect, so the doctor increased the dose very, very gradually. In three months, the patient was taking an effective dose for her condition.[9]

Some poor metabolizers need tiny doses. An 84-year-old woman suffered a prolonged depression after her husband died. Prozac helped a lot, but caused severe insomnia. Her doctor switched to the liquid and began with just one drop. With two drops, the depression faded. With three drops, the insomnia reappeared. Just two drops—less than 1 mg—was this woman's best dose, less than 5 percent of the 20-mg dose that is usually prescribed.

As our knowledge of pharmacogenetics gets adopted into everyday medicine, it will require doctors to use precision prescribing. But this will take years, maybe decades. Until then, you can obtain the same precision in your treatment by educating yourself about the precision-prescribing method and making your new knowledge part of your patient-doctor relationships.

6

Women and Seniors— Special Considerations With Statin Drugs

Cardiovascular disease is the leading killer among women, just as it is among men. According to an article in the *Archives of Internal Medicine*:

Cardiovascular disease, primarily coronary heart disease, outnumbers the next 16 causes of death (including all cancers) in women combined. Women are 4 to 8 times more likely to die of cardiovascular disease than of any other disease.[1]

WOMEN: WHY EXTRA CAUTION IS NEEDED WHEN STARTING STATINS

Traditionally, coronary disease has been considered less serious and, therefore, less vigorously treated in women. Younger women are at less cardiovascular risk than men, but after menopause women catch up in a hurry. "People tend to think of cardiovascular disease as a male affliction because the symptoms show up 10 years earlier in men," states Dr. Artemis Simopoulos, "but women catch up after menopause. In fact, on an annual basis, more women die from heart attacks than men. Five times more women die from a heart attack than from breast cancer."[2] Nevertheless, most women consider cancer their greatest health risk, whereas only a small percentage know that cardiovascular disease really is.

Today, experts recommend that postmenopausal women should be evaluated and treated for cholesterol disorders just as vigorously as men. But there can be a downside to this, as one woman wrote:

My doctor prescribed Lipitor to me. I checked it out, and it seemed safe. However, I had a bad reaction to it, and by the time my doctor was convinced Lipitor was the problem (it was the only thing I was taking), I was so ill it took over a year for me to recover.

This woman's doctor couldn't understand how the standard 10-mg starting dose of Lipitor could affect her so powerfully. But in fact, looking at her cholesterol levels, she needed only a 22 percent LDL-C reduction. This warranted only 2.5 mg of Lipitor initially. Instead, she got 10 mg—400 percent more. Because there is nothing in the package insert or PDR about 2.5 or 5 mg of Lipitor, many doctors think that 10 mg is the lowest effective dose of Lipitor and that's what they prescribe.

The fact is, this woman might have needed even less than 2.5 mg of Lipitor, because studies repeatedly show that women often respond to lower statin doses than men. In a study of Lipitor and Zocor, the dose requirements for women were less than for men.[3] Another study showed that equal doses of Zocor and Mevacor produced significantly higher blood levels in women than in men.[4] In a study of the now-banned Baycol, women taking 0.2 mg got nearly as much LDL-C reduction as men taking the full 0.4 dose.[5]

Some doctors have noticed that women can have problems with statins. At a conference, Dr. Sheldon Hendler, the author of the *Physicians' Desk Reference for Nutritional Supplements,* commented: "Many women are intolerant to statins."[6] This is not really surprising because, on average, women are smaller than men, and women outnumber men in the older age group. Women have a lower percentage of water and higher percentage of body fat, which may alter drug distribution. Because of a lower cardiac output, women generally have reduced blood flow to the liver and kidneys compared with men. There are also differences in the drug metabolizing enzymes in the intestine and liver.[7] All of these factors may alter the dynamics of statin utilization and elimination in women as compared to men.

Despite these facts, women are almost always prescribed the same powerful statin doses as men. Some women can handle these doses, but many women cannot. Because drug research has focused inadequately on this issue, the guidelines for doctors rarely mention gender as a factor to consider when selecting doses. That is why I published an article titled "Do Standard Doses of Frequently Prescribed Drugs Cause Preventable Adverse Effects in Women?" in the *Journal of the American Medical Women's Association (JAMWA),* and statins were one of the categories of medications I discussed at length.[8] Other researchers are also raising this issue:

For a number of drugs it is well recognized that women suffer more frequently from side-effects, however it is often not clear if this is due to gender differences in the pharmacokinetics [drug metabolism in the body] or pharmacodynamics [how drugs affect the body]. Very little is known about these gender-related differences and the possibility that women may show a different pattern of treatment response than men.[9]

In 2001, we began to understand why standard drug doses are too strong for millions of women. That year a report by the U.S. General Accounting Office revealed that only 22 percent of the subjects in early studies for establishing the doses of new medications were women. Because 78 percent of subjects were men, the doses derived from these studies were suitable for men—and often excessive for women. Worse, even when dose differences between the genders were identified, these differences were largely ignored and not reflected in the prescribing guidelines for doctors.[10] Thus, women continue getting the same strong medication doses as men and continue to suffer more side effects.[11]

A 2001 report by the National Academy of Sciences explained why the problem continues to persist. The report showed that in many areas of medical research, men are still viewed as the norm. Gender differences are overlooked or under-reported, downplaying rather than highlighting gender differences.[12] Commenting on this report, Dr. Raymond Woosley, Vice President of Health Services at the University of Arizona, stated that many drug studies he sees "don't consider sex differences at all."[13]

Such methods create extra risks for women, who need medications to prevent and treat cardiovascular disease as much as men do. Yet women are not prescribed statins nearly as often as men.[14] This general undertreatment is then compounded by overtreatment when statins are actually prescribed, because many women receive statin doses that are unnecessarily strong and trigger preventable side effects.

How important is this issue for women? Women have more chronic diseases, see doctors more often, and take more medications than men.[14] In the U.S., 55 percent of women take a prescription drug daily versus 37 percent of men.[15] Moreover, women account for more of the older population than men. Women comprise 67 percent of those over age 65, and this population has more medical disorders and takes more medication than any other. And women predominate even more among people in their eighties and nineties, the most medication-sensitive and at-risk population of all. Given the statistics, perhaps drug research should treat women as the norm instead of men. Better yet, maybe it should recognize the differences and develop drug doses to fit all sizes, ages, and genders.

Tailoring drug doses for women is especially important with statins not only because some women respond to lower statin doses, but also because the overall benefits of statins are not as well established for women as for men.[16] This may be because of the populations in which statins have been studied or because women get heart disease later than men, but until this issue is clarified, it is important to avoid unnecessarily aggressive statin therapy that may produce greater risks than benefits for many women. Moreover, because it appears that for women, a low HDL-C level may be a more important risk factor for developing cardiovascular disease than a high LDL-C level, statins may not be the best choice for some women.

SENIORS AND STATINS

Side effects hit seniors the hardest. Seniors make up just 19 percent of the American population, yet 39 percent of medication-related hospitalizations and 51 percent of medication-related deaths occur in the elderly.[17] The hospital is no refuge: hospital patients have a 30 percent chance of a medication reaction, and the risk is even greater for the elderly.[11] *The New England Journal of Medicine* states:

> The overall incidence of adverse drugs reactions in the elderly is two to three times that found in young adults. Furthermore, the incidence is probably underestimated.[18]

One reason that seniors have such a high incidence of adverse reactions is that seniors require more medications: 79 percent of seniors take at least one prescription drug daily versus 46 percent of the general population. The average senior takes three prescription drugs and at least one nonprescription drug a day. This multi-medication use adds to seniors' risks: with two or more drugs, the chances of an adverse interaction are estimated at 30 percent.[11] The risk increases with the number of drugs, and many seniors take five or seven or nine drugs daily.

Still, many medication reactions in seniors could be avoided by using the very lowest, effective doses of drugs. "In the elderly, and especially in people over 75 or 80, I often use doses that are so low, they are almost homeopathic," one internist told me. Yet today, more and more drugs are marketed with the exact same doses for seniors and young adults. Fewer and fewer drugs are designed for the special sensitivities, smaller size, greater frailty, multiple illnesses, and multiple-medication usage of seniors.

If there ever was a population that warranted precision prescribing, it is seniors. With children we adjust many drug doses for age and size, but we do so much less frequently for seniors. Yet we know that seniors metabolize drugs more slowly than younger people, so they develop higher and more prolonged drug levels—which correlates with seniors' higher incidence of side effects. We know that seniors' tissues are often more sensitive and their systems less resilient to the potent effects of drugs. Nevertheless, these basic facts are all too often ignored by drug companies, and the guidelines they provide to doctors all too often fail to suggest special attention for seniors. Gerontologists everywhere stress the importance of using extra caution and the lowest effective doses in the elderly (see the quotes on page 78), but doing so is becoming increasingly difficult even for aware doctors because so many drugs are marketed as one-size-fits-all.

One of the reasons that Dr. Graveline (see Chapter 1) reacted severely to Lipitor is that he was 70 years old and Lipitor rises to substantially higher blood levels in older people. The Lipitor package insert tells doctors that Lipitor produces "a greater degree of LDL-lowering at any dose in the elderly patient population compared to younger adults."[19] So seniors should get less Lipitor, right? Yes, but instead they get the same strong Lipitor doses as younger people. Statin doses are the same for young and old even when we know that statin levels rise significantly higher in seniors. Mevacor blood levels rise 45 percent in seniors versus young adults, yet the manufacturer's standard starting doses are the same. Plasma levels of Pravachol rise 27 percent higher in elderly men versus younger men, and 46 percent in elderly women versus younger women. A 46 percent increase is enough for many other drugs to be recommended at lower doses for elderly patients, but not with Pravachol.[19] Remember, these numbers are averages; many older people get much higher blood levels, but drug research concerns itself with statistics, not individuals.

In fact, the manufacturers' recommended doses for every statin are identical for seniors and young adults. Not one suggests special consideration for seniors in their dosage guidelines, not even for people over 80. This includes even Crestor, the newest and most potent statin. No wonder the side-effect epidemic is not slowing down.

The fact that drug company-recommended doses are the same whether you are very old, frail, or taking multiple medications defies medical science and common sense. Studies repeatedly demonstrate that seniors respond to lower, safer statin doses,[20–23] but when the dosage guidelines in package inserts and the PDR do not suggest this obvious option, doctors do not consider it. Most doctors have never seen the studies showing that seniors can respond to lower doses. Doctors assume that the drug companies and FDA have been thorough and that their guidelines are beyond

Experts Recommend Lower Doses for Older People

Older people can be especially sensitive to the effects of powerful medications. This is why medical journal articles and reference books recommend a start-low go-slow approach.

■ *Journal of the American Geriatrics Society:* "Choosing the correct dose of a drug therapy is critical when prescribing for older people because adverse effects are often dose-related. The conventional wisdom has been to 'start low and go slow.'"[27]

■ *Goth's Medical Pharmacology:* "In general the best approach is to start with lower doses and to increase dosage slowly and in small increments."[28]

■ **Public Citizen's** *Worst Pills, Best Pills II:* "If drug therapy is indicated, in most cases it is safer to start with the dose which is lower than the usual adult dose."[29]

■ *Archives of Internal Medicine:* "The elderly are especially sensitive to both the intended pharmacologic effects of drugs and their undesirable adverse reactions."[30]

■ *British Medical Journal (BMJ):* "If drug treatment is necessary, the lowest feasible dose of the drug should be used."[31]

reproach, so doctors usually follow them faithfully, inflexibly. But you don't have to agree. An 83-year old woman heard me speak and, when her doctor prescribed Lipitor, insisted on starting with half a pill (5 mg). Her LDL-C dropped from 140 to 82 mg/dl, a reduction of 41 percent.

Side effects can be prevented in seniors, just as they can be prevented in most people. Most side effects are dose-related, so preventing side effects means starting low and going slow, which is particularly important in seniors. Indeed, despite some of its questionable decisions, the FDA agrees in principle:

There is evidence that older adults tend to be more sensitive to drugs than younger adults, due to their generally slower metabolisms and organ functions. . . . The old adage, 'Start low and go slow,' applies especially to the elderly.[24]

If you are elderly, ask your doctor about starting with a lower, safer, proven-effective statin dose. Moreover, because recent evidence suggests that lipoprotein A is an important risk factor for vascular disease, stroke, and death in seniors,[25,26] a niacin derivative might be preferred over a statin if you are older, male, and have an elevated level of lipoprotein A.

7

Effective Strategies for Dealing with Side Effects and Other Problems with Statins

There is no question that these drugs are miracle drugs. They save millions of lives every year. What irks me, is it's important to know all sides of the equation, and nobody's paying attention to the toxic side of the equation.[1]

—CARDIOLOGIST PAUL PHILLIPS, MD

American doctors are among the best-trained doctors in the world. The majority care about their patients and make great efforts to treat them properly. Yet, though the discovery of statins has allowed doctors to reduce the risks of cardiovascular disease for millions of people, there is a lot of important information about statin side effects that is not well known among doctors or patients. This makes it difficult to make the right decisions when side effects occur. The result is frustrated doctors and unhappy patients who quit treatment.

The majority of people tolerate statins pretty well, but many others suffer side effects. More than half of the people who start on statins quit treatment within a year, and after a few years, only about 25 percent remain on the drugs.[2] "Most statin users get side effects, usually muscle discomfort or gastrointestinal problems that do not seem to diminish with time," a pharmacist told me. "Eventually, most of them discontinue their medication." This is regrettable because most statin side effects can be handled easily without people having to stop their medication. All of the common side effects with statins are dose-related. This means they are preventable by using the precision-prescribing method that matches statin doses to each person's need and tolerance. Unfortunately, most doctors are not taught how to do this. Although medical students' courses in pharmacology discuss individual variation in drug response as a general principle, few courses actually teach students how to individualize treatment with specific drugs.

Nationally recognized experts have repeatedly expressed concern about the gaps in the information doctors receive in medical school and beyond about medications. Dr. Jerry Avorn of the Harvard School of Public Health warned:

> There is an informational void about pharmaceuticals in the training of most doctors, despite the importance of the prescription in medical care. . . . Most of those who have looked thoughtfully at this process have been appalled at its inadequacy.[3]

According to Dr. Raymond L. Woosley, Vice President of Health Services, University of Arizona, and former Chairman of Pharmacology at Georgetown University:

> Only about fifteen of the medical schools today teach formal courses in clinical pharmacology, which is the discipline that emphasizes interindividual variability in response to drugs. This small effort will never counter the overwhelming message from the drug industry that one dosage is all that is needed and everyone will respond nicely without side effects.[4]

Moreover, few doctors are taught how to recognize, interpret, and deal with medication side effects. A report of the U.S. Department of Health and Human Services found that *only 16 percent* of clerkship programs for medical students included formal lectures about adverse drug events.[5] The result is that the serious impact of minor side effects is often overlooked. The only minor side effect is someone else's side effect. Muscle aches, abdominal pain, flatulence, or memory lapses may be minor compared to the life-threatening diseases healthcare professionals deal with every day, but minor side effects can still make people miserable and disrupt normal functioning. A study in the *Journal of General Internal Medicine* found that minor side effects occur frequently in everyday medical practice and that many doctors do not deal with them effectively. The study concluded: "Physicians often take these types of reactions for granted in the course of medical therapy. However, it is important to realize that these events are not minor to patients; physicians may underestimate the impact of these events on patient satisfaction, healthcare utilization, and quality of life."[6] When this happens, patients lose trust and forgo treatment.

The whole healthcare system tends to downplay the problems with medications. "Adverse events that do not pose a severe threat to the patient's health and are, therefore, considered nonserious are understudied in pharmacotherapy," stated an article in *Pharmacotherapy*. "Such events are seldom systematically assessed, and frequency figures are usually not reliable."[7] Regarding statins, cardiologist Paul Phillips adds, "Talking about the side effects remains a touchy subject in the medical community. The drugs [statins] can make such a profound difference in cholesterol levels and risk for heart attack and stroke that cardiologists don't want patients to be afraid to take them."[8]

There is nothing wrong with emphasizing the positive, but doing so strikes a false chord when side effects occur and doctors fail to acknowledge or deal with them. When doctors do not recognize and find solutions for side effects, patients do not put up with it for long. This is a major reason that so many people stop treatment with statins. This is why I say that *even minor side effects can have major consequences*. When minor statin side effects drive patients from treatment, the result can be catastrophic: premature heart attacks, strokes, and death. That is not minor.

Statin drugs can be extremely helpful—but only if side effects are prevented or, if they occur, solved. Here are six effective strategies for handling problems that commonly occur with statin drugs. These strategies can help you to avoid side effects, such as muscle pain, memory loss, and abdominal discomfort. If you are already experiencing side effects, these strategies can help you and your doctor handle them effectively, so that treatment can continue. The quick and effective handling of problems caused by statins can result in a win-win situation, not only for patients and doctors, but also for the entire healthcare system.

1. MAKING SURE A STATIN SIDE EFFECT IS NOT IGNORED

After being placed on 10 mg of Lipitor, a woman developed constant muscle and joint pain, which she reported to her physician. "My doctor swears my symptoms cannot be from the medication. I stopped the medication anyway. In two weeks, my energy returned to normal and the pain improved. It is now a month after last taking the drug. Still some mild elbow pain and hand pain, but my energy level is high again and pain improves every day. I have also lost about five pounds—simply from being able to move around again, clean house, walk my dog."

The PDR not only lists muscle pain (myalgia) as a statin side effect, it also contains a special warning section about muscle breakdown and acute muscle degeneration (a medical emergency) with all statins. Muscle pain, joint pain, stomach problems, and fatigue are common statin side effects that, according to patients, are commonly overlooked by their doctors. What is going on?

Many doctors are concerned and helpful when patients get side effects, but others have difficulty admitting that their drugs can do harm. My belief is that some doctors over-identify with their medications and lapse into psychological denial when patients report side effects. Other times, it is simply a matter of inadequate training or inadequate knowledge about statin side effects. The associate dean of one medical school told the *Wall Street Journal* of a medical resident whose patient had complained of muscle pain while on Lipitor and then on Pravachol. "The doctor thought the patient was probably nutty," the dean said, "until we told him it was a recognized syndrome."[8]

Dr. Andrew Herxheimer, of the highly respected Cochrane Centre in Britain, advises doctors:

> An unexplained disturbing event must be taken as the equivalent of a yellow traffic light: as a signal to proceed with caution and be prepared to stop. If the patient thinks the drug has caused the problem, it very often has. Patients should be routinely asked for their opinion.[9]

My experience matches Dr. Herxheimer's, but few doctors are trained to think this way. The results can be devastating. Health journalist Jane Brody wrote of an eighty-two-year-old Kansas woman who died from "long-standing but undetected muscle disease caused by a statin she'd taken for years."[10] For the entire time, the woman had complained of muscle pains that her doctors never related to the drug, even though muscle pain is one of the most common statin side effects. Why was this woman's side effect ignored? Somehow, many doctors have come to believe that unless a blood test for muscle damage is positive, the muscle or joint pain cannot be from the statin. Here is another example from a letter that appeared in the *People's Pharmacy* column:

> My husband has taken a number of cholesterol-lowering medicines during the last several years, including Lipitor, Zocor and Pravachol. Each time, he experiences muscle pain and weakness and has to stop the medicine. The doctor does a blood test and insists the drug is not responsible. But when my husband stops the medicine, his pain dis-

appears. He is now on Crestor. In one month, it has lowered his cholesterol from 320 to 194, but he has a lot of pain in his shoulders and upper arms. He also has experienced memory problems, especially with names. Could these problems be related to the medicine?[11]

It takes a really closed mind to fail to observe that this man's muscle pain is directly attributable to statin drugs. Medical science acknowledges that when an adverse effect occurs with a drug, then disappears when the drug is stopped, then reappears when the drug is started again, it is pretty definite proof of a medication-related problem. I will discuss this further when I explain the Side-Effect Probability Scale later in this chapter. You can use the information found in this scale to your advantage when trying to convince obstinate doctors of the obvious.

Why are doctors so resistant to admitting that statins might have some adverse qualities? All drugs have unintended effects. Even the most beneficial drug can cause harm in some people. This is basic medical science. So how doctors came to believe otherwise about statins is not certain, but I suspect it has to do with the intense marketing and invariably positive spin about statins from drug companies and their 90,000 sales representatives to doctors' offices. Dr. Phillips was one of the thousands of doctors turning a deaf ear when his patients complained about muscle pain with statins. "They would come in aching, and I would say, 'Shut up and take your statin.'" Finally, Dr. Phillips began questioning the accepted wisdom. He has now conducted a study showing that muscle pain frequently occurs without positive blood tests for muscle injury.[8]

Cardiologist Stephen Sinatra states, "People can experience symptoms such as muscle fatigue and soreness on statins without registering any enzymatic changes."[12] This is important because, according to Dr. Sinatra, much of the muscle pain can be ameliorated with coenzyme Q_{10}. Unfortunately, many doctors are not aware of this. Coenzyme Q_{10}, a natural product, cannot be patented, so it has no profit value to drug companies and, therefore, is not mentioned in their marketing.

A serious secondary problem that frequently occurs when side effects are not properly identified is the *prescribing cascade*.[13] As described by side-effect expert Jerry Gurwitz, MD, who, with Paula Rochon, MD, coined the term:

. . . [The prescribing cascade] begins when an adverse drug event is misinterpreted as a new medical condition. Another drug is then prescribed, and the patient is placed at risk of developing additional adverse effects relating to potentially unnecessary treatment.[14]

Statin-triggered muscle pain can lead to a prescription for muscle relaxants, which can cause lethargy or weakness. Muscle or joint pain can lead to the use of anti-inflammatory drugs, which can cause stomach pain, depression, or ringing in the ears; long-term usage can result in gastric hemorrhage or kidney damage.

The prescribing cascade is seen with many other drugs besides statins. Very commonly, doctors prescribe dependency-causing anti-anxiety drugs or sleep remedies for the agitation and insomnia provoked by Prozac, Zoloft, Paxil, and other top-selling antidepressants. These side effects are also dose-related, so the solution is precision prescribing, not more drugs.

What You Can Do

If your doctor does not recognize a common statin side effect, it is up to you. If the side effect is painful or appears serious, do not wait. Check the information in the package insert that came with the drug, or refer to medical references such as the PDR. Pharmacists can provide drug information, including package inserts or lists of known side effects. You can also obtain package inserts through an online search of the drug. Drug information is also accessible through the websites of the manufacturer, the FDA, and mainstream medical institutions like Johns Hopkins Medical School, the Mayo Clinic, and the Cleveland Clinic. In fact, you can report your own side effect to the FDA by filling out the form found at *www.fda.gov/medwatch/safety/3500.pdf.*

An excellent online resource for researching the medical literature is *www.PubMed.org,* a search engine maintained by the National Institutes of Health. You can look up a word, combination of words, or an author. You can also get the abstracts of medical journal articles there. If you are not familiar with PubMed, many librarians can show you the basics. You can also get helpful information and a free electronic newsletter from my website—*www.MedicationSense.com* There are many other websites that offer good information about alternative, non-drug therapies. Here are a few: the American College for the Advancement of Medicine at *www.ACAM.org,* the American Holistic Medical Association at *www.holisticmedicine.org,* and the National Center for Complementary and Alternative Medicine of the National Institutes of Health at *http://nccam.nih.gov/.* Also, many of the doctors mentioned in this book who practice alternative medicine have informative websites worth viewing.

You can also call the drug company that manufactures your statin. Drug companies have consumer information lines for inquiries about their drugs. You can get their telephone numbers from directory assistance or in the first section of the PDR. Be sure to tell them of your reaction to their drug. They are required to keep records of such reports and relay them to the FDA.

However, none of these sources offers information on precision prescribing or the lower, safer doses I have written about in this book. Few of these mainstream sources will provide any information about natural alternatives. But as far as getting information about a common side effect, these sources should do.

If you find information about your side effect from one of these respected resources, take the evidence to your doctor. Doctors are trained to respect evidence-based information. Good doctors will look at any scientifically sound information. If your doctor refuses, find a better doctor.

---

2. Verifying a Side Effect That is Not Listed in the Package Insert or PDR

I've had lots of memory/mind problems on 10 mg of Lipitor. My doctor refuses to believe that it could be the drug, even though the problems went away when I took myself off of the stuff. I keep seeing more and more people on the web with the same problems. I printed out some of the descriptions and showed my doctor, but again she said there were no studies showing these side effects and these reports mean nothing.

You may run into particular difficulty getting your doctor's attention if you experience a side effect that is not listed in the package insert or PDR. Many doctors are not aware that the information found in package inserts is based on just a few studies done before drugs are approved by the FDA. Dr. Janet Woodcock, Director of the FDA's Center for Drug Evaluation and Research, told the *Los Angeles Times*, "The sad truth is that, even after all the clinical development that occurs with every drug and even after drugs have been approved for a time, we only have a crude idea of what they do in people."[15]

There are many important side effects that are not listed in package inserts or the PDR. A great deal of important new information is learned after drugs are approved and used by millions of people, but this new information may never appear in the PDR or it may take years getting there. Only 5 percent of serious side effects ever get reported to the FDA, and only 1 to 2 percent of so-called minor side effects; so even common side effects may never get reported enough to gain official attention. Even when a large number of side effects is reported, there is no routine, expeditious method for incorporating the information into package inserts or the PDR unless it is very serious or lethal. Thus, the lists in package inserts and the PDR are usually incomplete and outdated. However, many doctors assume the information has been updated for each yearly edition of the PDR. Most drug write-ups have not. It can take years or decades, if ever, for a newly recognized side effect to get added to package inserts and the PDR. There is no law requiring manufacturers to add information for minor side effects.

This is why doctors must pay attention to patients' complaints, because patients' reports are often the first signs of previously unrecognized side effects. As two experts put it, "The research data lags behind—rather than leads—experience in everyday clinical practice."[16] Everyday practice is the arena where many new drug toxicities are first discovered—by patients. Although encountering unlisted side effects should not surprise any doctor, unfortunately, many doctors are reluctant to make a diagnosis of a new side effect if it has not been reported previously.

Statin-related memory deficits are a perfect example. For years, evidence has been mounting that statins can impair cognitive and memory functioning, yet many statin package inserts do not list cognitive problems or forgetfulness among their side effects. These reactions may be subtle, but they can also be very serious. Older patients frequently worry that they are developing Alzheimer's or have had a stroke. The *People's Pharmacy* column has offered many examples of these problems with statins. Here is one:

Last fall my doctor prescribed Lipitor. After several months I found I was having trouble remembering names and coming up with the right word. At dinner once, I said,'Please pass the elephant,' though I wanted the bread. I told my husband that I thought I'd had a stroke. In January, a friend came to visit. She was worried about her memory and couldn't think of her daughter's name on the telephone. She too was on Lipitor. I asked my doctor to prescribe a different cholesterol medicine. Within a couple of weeks I was more mentally alert. But my friend (still on Lipitor) was in worse shape and afraid she would lose her job. Her doctor said forgetfulness could not be due to the drug. She finally stopped taking Lipitor and now is much sharper.[17]

These memory problems went away after discontinuing the statin, but it has been reported that, in some cases, memory or psychological symptoms persist. That is why it is not only important to recognize the reaction, but to do so quickly. Moreover, side effects that impair cognitive functioning can create risks that affect more than the patient. Recently, a flight surgeon wrote to me about Zocor impairing pilots' ability to perform complicated tasks and, therefore, creating a potential hazard for the pilots and their passengers. Dr. Duane Graveline, who runs a website (*www.spacedoc.net*) on statin reactions and has recently published *Lipitor, Thief of Memory*, reports hearing similar stories from pilots.

Dr. Beatrice Golomb, who is conducting a study supported by the National Institutes of Health on memory problems related to statins, told the *Wall Street Journal* that cognitive and memory problems "are substantially more common than one would divine from reading the [medical] literature." From her own vast experience in evaluating such cases, Dr. Golomb says that about 15 percent of patients develop some cognitive problem related to statin use. Yet, within the healthcare community, she states, "there are still people who are persuaded . . . that there are no cognitive effects from statins."[18] One of these people is Dr. Art Ulene, the prominent television and radio doctor and former family physician, who developed confusion, disorientation, and memory impairment. Ulene was diagnosed with transient global amnesia from a statin. This is the same problem that Dr. Graveline developed (see Chapter 1). Several weeks later, on statins again, Dr. Ulene developed severe muscle pain. These experiences have changed Dr. Ulene's perspective on these so-called miracle drugs.[19]

What You Can Do

If your side effect is not listed in the package insert or PDR, conduct your own search using the sources listed above. In addition, for some drugs, such as Lipitor, there are internet groups that can provide specific information about side effects. But be selective. The more scientific the information, the better. And do not be intimidated. Medical science has a method for determining the likelihood of a medication reaction even if it has not been reported elsewhere. The Side-Effect Probability Scale (page 89) describes how side effects can be categorized as definite, probable, possible, or unlikely.[20] For example, a side effect is considered *probable* if a patient develops symptoms after starting a medication, if the medical disorder or other factors are not likely causes of the symptoms, and if the symptoms abate when the drug is reduced or stopped. Under these circumstances, the medication is the probable cause, even if the side effect is not listed in the package insert, PDR, or elsewhere. The problem is, most doctors have never heard of the side-effect probalility scale. Yet, these scales are powerful tools used by researchers, academicians, and doctors who are publishing case reports in medical journals. This scale can be a powerful tool for you, too, if you experience a side effect that is not listed in standard sources of medical information.

Unfortunately, standard side-effect scales don't offer a category into which new side effects fit neatly. To fit the definite, probable, or possible categories, this type of scale requires a "recognized" reaction. New side effects have not been recognized previously, yet they may fit all of the other criteria of a definite or probable reaction. My feeling is that if a reaction develops after starting a new drug, cannot be explained by the illness or other factors, and abates with discontinuance of the drug, it is a *probable* adverse reaction.

In an optimal medical system, it would not be so difficult to get quick and helpful attention when you develop a side effect, even if it is not listed in standard resources. Many important medical discoveries began with simple observations in doctors' offices. "All science is rooted in observations," wrote Dr. Robert Brodell in *Postgraduate Medicine.* "Full-time physicians are in an ideal position to observe unusual cases, develop rational explanations for the findings, and follow progress to determine if their hypotheses appear to be valid."[21] Science does not begin and end with the drug industry research. Indeed, it is a notoriously known fact that drug company studies often fail to identify many common side effects in everyday practice. Sexual dysfunctions with Prozac, Zoloft, and similar drugs are notoriously downplayed in package inserts, while practitioners agree that 50 percent or more of patients develop sexual dysfunctions with these drugs.[22-24] The heart valve deformities and lethal pulmonary hypertension that caused the withdrawal of the weight-loss sensations Redux and Fen-Phen were not discovered in the manufacturer's studies, but by an alert lab technician, who had difficulty convincing her supervising doctors.

When former FDA commissioner David Kessler was asked about our system's failure to identify many serious side effects, he replied, "The real issue, probably more important than the system, is for people to be looking, to be on guard, to be looking for possible associations of drugs with reactions."[25] Research has shown that when doctors take an active role in identifying side effects, they find far more of them, which then allows them to adjust doses or drugs, and to keep their patients happy and in treatment. Dr. Sinatra states, "Nine times out of ten, patients will ascribe vague symptoms like weakness and aching to the process of growing older and not think to mention them, so it's up to us doctors to tease this out."[12]

At one of my recent lectures, a woman said that she had been in a statin study. "I began having trouble remembering things and sometimes I felt disconnected from my body. I thought I was losing it." This is known as

Side-Effect Probability Scale

Side-effect scales for evaluating medication side effects are widely accepted in academic medicine and frequently cited in studies and case reports in the medical literature. All medication reactions should be reported to the FDA's Medwatch program. The form is one page, easy to fill out, and accessible via the internet at *www.fda.gov/medwatch/safety/3500.pdf.*

■ *Definite* **Adverse Drug Reaction**
1. Occurred within reasonable proximity of taking a drug.
2. A recognized reaction to the suspected drug.
3. Abated following withdrawal of the drug.
4. Recurred following re-exposure to the drug.
5. Could not be reasonably explained by the patient's condition or other factors.

Comment: In everyday practice, *definite* reactions are rarely seen because there are medical or ethical problems with re-exposing patients to drugs that may already have caused them side effects.

■ *Probable* **Adverse Drug Reaction**
1. Occurred within reasonable proximity of taking a drug.
2. A recognized reaction to the suspected drug.
3. Abated following withdrawal of the drug.
4. Could not be reasonably explained by the patient's condition or other factors.

Comment: Many adverse effects fall into the *probable* category. "Recognized reactions" include side effects listed in package inserts and the PDR, or in other drug references or medical journals.

■ *Possible* **Adverse Drug Reaction**
1. Occurred within reasonable proximity of taking a drug.
2. Possibly a recognized reaction to the suspected drug.
3. Abated following withdrawal of the drug.
4. Possibly explained by the patient's condition or other factors.

Comment: Sometimes it is difficult to differentiate a medication reaction from the symptoms of a disease. *Possible* reactions can fit either category, but suspicion falls on the drug if it is a previously recognized reaction and it abates following discontinuation.

■ *Doubtful* **Adverse Drug Reaction**
1. Occurred within reasonable proximity of taking a drug.
2. Possibly a recognized reaction to the suspected drug.
3. More likely explained by the patient's condition or other factors.

Comment: *Doubtful* reactions are more likely explained by the medical condition or other factors. However, if the cause of the reaction remains unclear, discontinuing the drug may clarify its role in the symptoms.

derealization, a psychiatric symptom that can occur with drugs affecting the brain. She told the doctors and nurses running the study, but they insisted the drug could not cause it. After the study ended and the drug was stopped, it took months for the symptoms to abate, and ten months later the woman was still shaken by the experience. "I thought I was losing my mind. I still get upset thinking about it. It's good to finally know that it wasn't me, but the drug." If other researchers respond similarly when patients complain of problems, no wonder the side effect data is so inaccurate and the lists in package inserts and the PDR are incomplete.

On the other hand, when doctors are meticulous about inquiring and evaluating possible side effects, they help patients and medical science at the same time. This is important, because even when drug companies conduct exemplary studies, some adverse effects are going to be missed. For example, it is well known that side effects that occur in every 1 of 1,000 patients are often not identified in drug studies; but when 20 million people are taking the drug, it means that approximately 20,000 people are sustaining the side effects each year. Thus, the integrity of the entire system depends on doctors listening to their patients, and on your doing your homework and bringing your findings to your doctor.

3. DEALING WITH SIDE EFFECTS FROM STANDARD INITIAL STATIN DOSES

Julia is a fifty-seven-year-old woman with mildly elevated cholesterol and C-reactive protein levels. To reduce these, her doctor prescribed Lipitor at the standard 10-mg dose. Julia immediately experienced gastric irritation, abdominal cramps, and malaise. "This isn't worth it," Julia told me.

Abdominal discomfort and malaise are common side effects with statins, and they are dose-related. Moreover, the quick development of these side effects was indicative of a typical *first-dose reaction*, strongly suggesting that the standard dose of Lipitor was too strong for Julia. First-dose reactions are not really surprising when you consider that the drug industry and FDA employ a middle-dose approach for selecting drug doses.[26] A middle-dose derived from statistical averages is guaranteed to be too strong for 30 to 50 percent of patients.

First-dose reactions are a big problem with many types of medications. These problems could be avoided by starting with the lowest, proven-effective doses of drugs, but drug manufacturers like to keep dosing simple, so they do not produce these lower doses or mention them in package inserts or the PDR. When doctors prescribe the lowest doses in the PDR, they think they are prescribing the very lowest, safest, effective doses, but they are not. Julia's doctor undoubtedly thought he was prescribing the lowest, safest dose of Lipitor, because 10 mg is the lowest dose the manufacturer makes, and there is no mention of the effectiveness of 2.5 mg or 5 mg of Lipitor in the package insert, PDR, or other drug references.

What You Can Do

Show your doctor Table 3.1 (page 42) when a statin is being considered. Start with a dose that fits your LDL-C-reduction requirement. You may want to start even lower, because some people get even better responses than the averages, especially if they adopt a heart-healthy diet. If the lower dose is not strong enough, it can be gradually increased. No matter which dose you choose, if you develop side effects, reduce it further. You may be particularly medication-sensitive to this statin. Your doctor may want to switch you to another statin, and that is okay– as long as you start with a very low dose that is unlikely to trigger more side effects.

4. AVOIDING EXCESSIVE ATTENTION TO CHOLESTEROL LEVELS AND INADEQUATE ATTENTION TO PATIENT

Within three days of starting 10 mg of Lipitor, Marlene, a healthy, active sixty-four-year old, became increasingly dizzy and confused, fell down several steps, and required emergency care. These symptoms disappeared within forty-eight hours of stopping the drug. Marlene's doctor then prescribed a standard dose of Zocor, which caused side effects, and then Pravachol, which did the same. Fed up, Marlene quit treatment.

Marlene's cholesterol numbers were high, so the initial prescription of potent Lipitor was warranted. But once it became apparent that she was sensitive to statins, the need for a start-low go-slow approach was clear. Her doctor should have considered low doses of Zocor and Pravachol, but that is not what the dosage guidelines for these drugs recommend, so treatment failed again and again. Why? Marlene's treatment failed because it focused entirely on her cholesterol levels, and not enough on her body's ability to tolerate statin medication.

Marlene's well-meaning doctor, like most, was never taught that some people are sensitive to medications, especially potent ones like statins. Like most doctors, he never saw the studies showing that some people get much greater responses to statins than the averages. This information—the dose-response information so important for understanding individual variation—is not offered in most package inserts or PDR drug descriptions. And like most doctors, Marlene's doctor never stumbled across my writings on the effectiveness of lower, safer doses of statins. Marlene's doctor is not alone. He is in the vast majority. A pharmacist told me years ago, "If a medication does not work or causes side effects, most physicians just switch from one to another, then another, then another, until they either find a drug that works, or they or the patient give up. Very few physicians adjust drug doses to fit their patients. Most do not deviate from the drug company guidelines in the PDR." Dr. Herxheimer adds:

> Clinicians rarely think critically about the dose-response relations of the drugs they use. Many drugs have been introduced at doses that later were found to be too high; and usually years have passed, with unnecessary toxicity, before action is taken.[27]

So instead of using lower doses for this obviously statin-sensitive woman, Marlene's doctor followed the guidelines he had and provoked a series of preventable side effects, ultimately driving his patient from needed treatment. This was not his intention or desire, but it happened anyway—just as it happens in thousands of doctors' offices every day.

What You Can Do

Remind your doctor that according to the National Cholesterol Education Program, statin treatment guidelines "are intended to inform, not replace, the physician's clinical judgment, which must ultimately determine the appropriate treatment for each individual."[28] Your doctor's clinical judgment should always begin with an understanding of you and your medication tendencies. Patients should not be fitted to cookbook doses determined from averaged results in unrepresentative studies. Drugs and doses must be tailored to the specific needs and tolerances of individuals. As stated before, individual variation is the rule, not the exception. No matter which medication is being prescribed, doctors must always consider your unique characteristics. This is a basic medical principle, as reflected in medicine's most respected drug reference, *Goodman & Gilman's The Pharmacologic Basis of Therapeutics*:

It is no less crucial to have a scientific approach to the treatment of an individual patient than to use this approach when investigating drugs in a research setting.[29]

Indeed, we know that the results of drug research, which provide the average responses from carefully selected subjects, frequently do not apply to everyday office patients. Patients in doctors' offices are more diverse with many more complicating factors, such as other illnesses or other medications than the subjects who fit the strict, exclusionary criteria of drug studies. Therefore, applying a scientific approach with statins includes considering your age, size, use of other medications, state of health, and the mildness or severity of the condition being treated. It includes knowing your history of good responses or problems with medications, and your degree of medication sensitivity. It includes having knowledge of the full range of effective drug doses, especially the lower, safer statin doses that work.

5. Avoiding Excessive Dosing with Statins

Reported to the FDA: A forty-year old nurse with mild hypertension and a total cholesterol of 276 (LDL-C 150) was started on 40 mg of Zocor. After seven days, she began having difficulty breathing. The Zocor was stopped, but she died three months later from a rare lung disease (interstitial pulmonary fibrosis) that was attributed to the Zocor by her doctor and an independent medical examiner.[30]

The use of stronger and stronger initial statin doses is being seen more frequently each year. The result is that as drug companies have bumped their initial statin doses by 100 percent to 400 percent, millions of people are getting started at doses far beyond their LDL-reduction goals. For example, the manufacturer's recommended initial dose of Zocor was originally 10 mg; now it is 20 mg or 40 mg. Lipitor was 10 mg; now it is 10 mg, 20 mg, or 40 mg. Pravachol was originally 10 mg and 20 mg; now it is 40 mg. Unfortunately, this trend is accelerating. In 2003, Crestor was approved by the FDA with even greater potency at its 10 and 20 mg initial doses than any other statin. Subsequently, new studies showed that super-strong 80-mg Lipitor was superior to moderate-strength 40-mg Pravachol in slowing the development of atherosclerosis and in preventing complications and deaths in people with acute, severe coronary disease. These events are already leading to more aggressive statin treatment for people with coronary disease, which may be warranted if done carefully. But the downside is that doctors, many of whom have become overly enthusiastic about statins, may also be prescribing these super-strong doses to people with mild-to-moderate cholesterol elevations, resulting in overmedication and unnecessary side effects.

Minor side effects are not so minor to the people sustaining them. People will not put up with discomfort or impaired functioning for long, and they should not have to, especially when these problems can be so easily avoided with the precision-prescribing approach. Although serious side effects may be infrequent, they do happen and, therefore, must be considered when statin doses are chosen. Muscle degeneration, liver toxicity, and kidney failure—all dose-related—have been reported in hundreds of cases. Deaths have occurred. The higher the dose, the greater the risk.

The terminal pulmonary fibrosis in the case discussed earlier may be rare, but it has been linked to statins in reports in medical journals,[31–33] and rare reactions do happen to some people. This woman's LDL-C was not very high. She may not have needed statin therapy at all, but if she did, her LDL-C level indicated the use of just 5 mg of Zocor. But her doctor, overconfident about statins, like so many doctors, chose an excessive dose because he probably believed that statins are virtually harmless. This was an entirely avoidable tragedy.

Overconfidence among doctors is a big problem with statins. The quick embrace by doctors of every new, positive study while ignoring reports of adverse effects is very worrisome. In the study comparing super-strong Lipitor to moderate-strength Pravachol, doctors could hardly contain their elation with the superiority of the super-strong approach, yet they completely ignored the fact that the adverse liver effects were significantly higher in the super-strong Lipitor group. There is an element of selective thinking or cognitive dissonance going on here. Maybe it has been so long since doctors have had a new wonder drug, the temptation to view statins as such is overwhelming. One statin expert told me, "There are doctors who claim that no LDL-C level is too low, and no statin dosage, therefore, too aggressive."

Doctors' desire to reduce cardiovascular disease is praiseworthy. Their concerns about undertreatment are valid. However, this does not warrant the overtreatment of millions of people, a problem that will only worsen as 20 million more Americans are placed on statins for high cholesterol or elevated CRP. Statin therapy must be individualized. Precision prescribing is easily done and saves time and money in the long run. Other doctors share my concern, as reflected in this letter to *JAMA:*

The adverse effects of statins are a concern. Adverse effects will undoubtedly increase under the new guidelines as more people are treated. It might be advisable to determine the minimum statin dosage that provides cardioprotection. As with aspirin, this may be much lower than for other indications.[34]

A few weeks after I read about the nurse's death, my cousin called. His doctor had started him on Zocor. Based on my cousin's cholesterol levels, 20 mg was the proper initial dose, but the doctor prescribed 40 mg. I told him to take 20 mg; but even this caused side effects. Ultimately, he reduced the dose to 10 mg, which was still strong enough to achieve his LDL-C goal.

What You Can Do

Insist that the initial statin dose your doctor prescribes matches the LDL-C reduction you require according to Table 3.1 (page 42). If your condition is not severe, you can start even lower to see if you get a greater than average response. Many people do, especially if they also adopt a heart-healthy diet. If the lower dose is not enough, it can be gradually increased—this is the precision-prescribing method. The goal is to minimize the risks as you find the right statin dose for you.

The precision-prescribing method is not necessarily for everyone. If you do not want to take the time for a start-low go-slow approach, be sure that you are not prescribed a higher dose than your LDL-C reduction warrants. Remember, using statins should not be a one-step process. Getting the dose right means rechecking your cholesterol levels and adjusting the dosage if necessary. This is sometimes necessary even for people starting with standard doses or higher.

---

6. IDENTIFYING AND TREATING MEDICATION-SENSITIVE INDIVIDUALS

George was forty-seven years old when his doctor prescribed Mevacor. George's cholesterol was only moderately elevated, but the doctor followed the drug company guidelines and prescribed the standard initial dose, 20 mg. From prior experience, George knew he was sensitive to medications, so he split the pill and began with 10 mg. This provided such good LDL-C reduction, George was able to reduce the dose to 5 mg. His doctor was amazed.

Precision prescribing is not rocket science. It is common sense, which is just as important in medicine as it is in everyday life. The dosage guidelines in the Mevacor package insert and PDR state: "Patients requiring reductions in LDL of 20 percent or more to achieve their goal should be started on 20 mg/day of Mevacor." George needed a 20-percent reduction in LDL-C, so his doctor prescribed 20 mg. Yet, the package insert and PDR also contain a table showing that although 20 mg of Mevacor reduces LDL-C 27 percent on average, 10 mg reduces LDL-C 21 percent—just what George required.[35] So why do the manufacturer's guidelines recommend a 100 percent stronger dose?

No law requires doctors to follow manufacturers' guidelines. Doctors are expected to exercise their own judgment in selecting drugs and doses. Knowing that side-effect risks increase with higher doses, doctors should be wary about standard initial statin doses, especially for patients like George, who are willing to make dietary or other changes. Even though doctors have less time than ever to spend with patients, it is still a fundamental aspect of practicing medicine to assess each patient's characteristics and experiences with medications. It takes only a few seconds to ask, "Are you sensitive to medications? Have you had problems with side effects previously?" Why not give people with histories of reactions or a preference for emphasizing safety the opportunity to try a lower, proven-effective statin dose? The only way to see if you get a greater-than-average LDL-C reduction is to try a lower dose. Reducing cholesterol usually is not an emergency. There is time to start with a low dosage, see how you do, and proceed accordingly. There is time to place safety first.

Sometimes the fault lies with healthcare systems that shuffle patients to a new doctor with every visit. It is almost impossible for doctors to provide proper treatment without the ability to follow cases and make adjustments when indicated. Many types of medications—statins, antihypertensives, and antidepressants, for example—require follow-up to confirm whether the patient is improving or needs dose adjustments.

What You Can Do

Identify the right statin dose for you according to Table 3.1 (page 42), and ask your doctor to start you at that amount or a slightly lower dosage. For optimal care, choose, if possible, a healthcare system that allows continuity with the doctors you see. Once you find a doctor you like, you will not want to switch.

HOW TO DEAL EFFECTIVELY WITH YOUR DOCTOR ABOUT MEDICATIONS AND SIDE EFFECTS

Most doctors are dedicated, knowledgeable people who want to help their patients. Most doctors care. Yet, like all humans, they have their viewpoints and biases. Doctors are taught to trust the information they receive and to be skeptical of information from non-mainstream sources, especially if it is anecdotal or subjective. They are concerned that under-dosing can cause ineffective treatment. Most doctors have not seen much, if any, of the low-dose data. Drug companies are the main source of information for most doctors. These companies realize they can influence doctors' decisions by controlling the information they receive. So the drug industry floods doctors with advertising and offers "free" seminars on the unmatched benefits of their products. They also send out some 90,000 sales representatives to patrol doctors' offices, disperse free samples, and monitor doctors' prescribing practices via networks connected to pharmacies nationwide. With such dominance, other important information often has a hard time being heard. Thus, it can take years or decades for objective information to filter down to everyday practitioners. A lot of this good information never gets to doctors at all.

For example, nearly half of the doctors in America have never seen the low-dose guidelines of the national expert panel on hypertension, although this panel has published reports every five years for decades.[36] When the laboratory methods for measuring the effects of Coumadin (warfarin) changed, pushing people's Coumadin doses to toxic levels, it took decades for the word to reach the majority of doctors, despite repeated articles in top medical journals. Millions were seriously harmed and thousands died unnecessarily.[37]

Other examples abound, but the point is that there is a huge gap in the information that doctors receive, and most doctors do not realize it. This is why you must be informed yourself. Too many doctors get only part of the picture, and most of that picture is drawn by the drug industry; so it is no surprise that pills are their first solution for most medical problems. It is why doctors rely on the drug companies' dosage guidelines, even though studies have repeatedly shown that lower doses work. It is also why some doctors overlook side effects that have been repeatedly reported in medical journals.

If you want to be sure of getting the right statin drug and dosage for you, especially if you want to start with a lower dose, you will probably have to furnish some information for your doctor. If you experience a side effect that is not listed in the drug package insert or the PDR, you may have trouble convincing your doctor, unless you bring scientific information from another reliable source.

Discussing medication doses and side effects with a doctor can be dicey. With less time than ever for each patient, doctors feel pressured—the average doctor listens to patients for only twenty-three seconds before interrupting them. Regarding medications, doctors rightly consider themselves the experts, and choosing drugs and doses has historically been their exclusive domain. So unfortunately, some doctors get defensive, and a few get hostile, when patients question their methods when it comes to prescribing medications. Indeed, some doctors get huffy with pharmacists who question a drug or dosage, even though pharmacists are officially mandated to do so if they see a prescription that might be incorrect. Pharmacists have told me of doctors who have asked them heatedly, "Do you have a medical license? Did you go to medical school?"

If a doctor says something like this to you, do not get ruffled. Be prepared, stay calm, and answer directly, "Of course not, but I do have a brain, and I have learned to search the medical literature [or, package inserts, drug references, etc.]. Let me show you what I have found." If your doctor is not cooperative, you may have to get more direct: "I'm taking the medication, so I'd like to have some say in the matter," or "Isn't this a joint relationship?" In other words, say something that is challenging but not offensive. Stand your ground. Remember, you are the one taking the drug, taking the risks, and paying a lot of money for the privilege.

For many patients, this is uncharted—and uncomfortable—territory. One man, a highly successful executive and marathon runner, had developed memory problems. When I told him that his Lipitor and Neurontin were probably responsible, he was uncomfortable with the idea of telling his doctor. He told me, "I'm pretty forceful in most situations. In my work, I ask a lot of questions, hard questions when necessary. But with doctors, I feel out of my element. I know so little, I never know what to ask. I pretty much take what they tell me on faith. What if my doctor says the drugs are not the cause? Who am I to question? What do I know about drugs?"

Information is power. That is why it is so vital for you to become your own researcher. Just as people do a lot of research before going to a car dealership or stereo store, researching medical information can empower you in health situations. And, fortunately, if you bring sound information, most doctors will listen. Many, in fact, will be appreciative. Doctors are trained to respect good scientific information, like the information published in medical journals. You can use this to your advantage. By providing scientifically sound information, you are offering material in a form that doctors can respect—that reasonable doctors will respect. My goal in writing scientific, evidence-based books and articles is to facilitate this process by providing the type of information that doctors and medical experts respect. This book, with its hundreds of references, is an example.

Many patients bring information from newspapers, magazines, and the internet to their doctors, and they are disappointed when their doctors are skeptical of such sources. The better your sources of information, the better your chances of being heard. A friend, who was having chronic muscle pain while taking Lipitor but not getting far with her doctor, called me. I told her to take my book, show the doctor the references I listed on dose-related side effects with statins, and take any other information she could find from mainstream medical websites or medical journals. Shortly after, she told me:

> My doctor finally agreed to try a half dose of Lipitor because, he said, he could see that I'd done my homework and I brought him good information from respectable sources. He told me that many of his patients just like to gripe about having to take drugs they need, but they don't present any convincing information. They just want to complain. So my doctor and I agreed to try a half dose. My doctor was skeptical, but he was willing to compromise. My LDL-C level remained low, and the aching in my muscles disappeared. He was quite surprised, but willing to continue with the half dose.

You are paying the costs and taking the risks, so you have a right to ask why your doctor is selecting a specific statin at a specific dose. Are there lower doses that work? What is his source of information? Yes, you may be asking questions your doctor is not accustomed to, but we must begin asking doctors to explain their decisions, to think about their choices, to consider other sources of information and alternative methods that work. Some doctors may be taken aback, but some of them will thank you for making them think outside the box. For many doctors, practicing medicine is the most fulfilling when they are actually required to rethink the decisions they make and consider new, worthwhile ideas.

Besides, precision prescribing is not a foreign medical concept. Doctors already practice precision prescribing with drugs like digoxin, insulin, and thyroid medications, so applying the concept to other drugs like statins is not a huge leap. If you do your homework and bring good information to the consultation, you will be much more likely to get a favorable response.

In addition, you will be redefining the nature of your relationship with your doctor for the better. In fact, providing good information to doctors can have a cumulative effect. It can improve your care, as well as the care of others. Multiply this by thousands of people bringing new, objective information to their doctors, and the system will improve for everyone and for future generations. If we are to forge a better healthcare system in which side effects are no longer a major cause of death and disability, it must begin with us.

8

Effective Alternative Therapies for Reducing Cholesterol and Other Risk Factors

Precision prescribing means considering all reasonable possibilities for treatment. Indeed, in an optimal healthcare system, solutions for many disorders would begin with nutrition, then natural interventions, then pharmaceuticals. That is not the predominant model today, but natural therapies have gained an unprecedented role in many people's healthcare. In 2000, 150 million Americans spent $17 billion dollars on dietary supplements. However, in 2002, the U.S. Department of Health and Human Services reported that "most complementary and alternative modalities have not yet been scientifically studied and found to be safe and effective."[1] This is not surprising, considering that every time you turn on the TV or radio, there is another promotion for a new supplement to cure whatever ails you. The supplement market is an unregulated modern-day Wild West in which there are too many claims and too little science. It is easy to see what prompted the American Medical Association to declare: "There is little evidence to confirm the safety or efficacy of most alternative therapies."[2]

Even in the Old West, good things were happening amid the tumult, and it is in the alternative world that people are seeking natural solutions that are more physiologic and safer than prescription pharmaceuticals. The result is that there are now several natural remedies that are proven to reduce LDL-C and a few that raise the good HDL-C. However, because of the limited financial resources of their manufacturers and little interest among mainstream doctors and journals, studies on these natural products are far fewer than those on prescription statins. Placebo-controlled, double-blind studies are few, and there are hardly any long-term studies of these products' impact on morbidity and mortality. Still, the studies that exist have been promising, and clinical experience has often been rewarding.

Dr. Robert Rowen, a practitioner of integrative medicine in Santa Rosa, CA who is board certified in family practice and a fellow of the American Academy of Family Physicians, wrote to me:

> Regarding alternatives to statins, my brother is a good case in point. With a cholesterol of 230, his doctor tried to talk him into taking a statin. Instead, I recommended a standard dose of red yeast rice and guggulipid. His LDL cholesterol dropped 30 points. I rarely have to use statin drugs between red yeast, guggulipid, niacin, and dietary change. The only time statins may be useful is for familial hypercholesterolemia [a severe, genetic form of elevated cholesterol]. I have not written an original prescription for statin drugs ever.

Dr. Rowen isn't alone. Thousands of doctors in North and South America, Europe, and Asia use alternative therapies to lower cholesterol without resorting to prescription drugs. These methods may not be FDA approved, but this does not mean they might not work. Doctors use prescription drugs every day in ways that are not FDA approved, so why not consider using proven-effective natural alternatives for lowering cholesterol and CRP?

Some doctors are uncomfortable using natural alternatives because it means making decisions on less scientific data than for prescription drugs. But following patients' cholesterol and CRP levels can gauge the effectiveness of the natural alternative. For patients with moderate cholesterol or CRP elevations, the situation is not an emergency, so there's time to try natural, less expensive methods if this is what the patient desires. Medical science supports decisions by doctors that involve trying unorthodox yet reasonable methods in situations that warrant them. Using natural supplements can be a valid approach for you, but cholesterol and CRP levels should still be monitored.

RED YEAST RICE

Chinese red yeast rice has significant potential to reduce healthcare costs and contribute to public health by reducing heart disease risk in individuals with moderate elevations of circulating cholesterol levels.[3]

—JOURNAL OF ALTERNATIVE AND COMPLEMENTARY MEDICINE

This viewpoint is also reflected in the *Journal of the American Academy of Family Physicians*, which usually takes a very cautious approach regarding natural supplements, but did not hesitate to publish a study of red yeast rice for reducing cholesterol. The conclusion: "So far, Cholestin [a brand of red yeast rice] has proved to be a cost-saving lipid-lowering medication."[4] Red yeast rice has been used in China since 800 A.D. It is produced by fermenting rice with a yeast (*Monascus purpurus*) that gives it a reddish hue. Red yeast rice contains approximately ten compounds that are similar to prescription statins, particularly lovastatin, the statin in Mevacor. Thus, for doctors who are adamant about obtaining statin-like effects, red yeast rice is a good alternative.

Yet some doctors are not impressed. One told me, "I look at it as a watered down version of Mevacor, so I don't use it." If he wants a statin-like effect, he said, he prescribes a statin, because the studies of effectiveness are far more extensive and the production of statins, regulated by the FDA, is guaranteed to deliver a standardized amount in each pill.

On the other hand, red yeast rice does not seem to cause the typical side effects—muscle pain, abdominal discomfort, liver irritation—that commonly occur with statins. Dr. Allan Magaziner, an alternative practitioner in Cherry Hill, NJ, and president of the American College for the Advancement of Medicine (ACAM), told me:

> I have used red yeast rice in more than five hundred patients, and it is remarkably effective. It is also very well tolerated. No muscle aches or pains. No liver enzyme elevations. It doesn't appear to lower coenzyme Q_{10} levels, although I have patients take a little CoQ_{10} for safety anyway. Red yeast rice does contain statin-like compounds, but I suspect that because it contains small amounts of multiple compounds, no one of them is large enough to produce problems.

Dr. Magaziner uses red yeast rice for people with moderate cholesterol elevations in the 200 to 260 range. He obtains LDL-C reductions of 20 percent to 25 percent and small increases in HDL-C. Some people get even better results. "I've seen some great results that are usually apparent within two months, sometimes within weeks," Dr. Magaziner told me. "Red yeast rice is my first choice for lowering cholesterol levels."

The usual dose of red yeast rice is 1,200 mg twice-daily. According to Dr. David Heber, a nutrition expert at UCLA and author of *What Color Is Your Diet*, a daily dose of red yeast rice contains about 5 mg of lovastatin. Dr. Magaziner sometimes starts with 1,200 mg once daily, then increases the dose if necessary. In recalcitrant cases, he adds another cholesterol-lowering supplement, policosanol. Scientific studies support Dr. Magaziner's findings. Studies in China have demonstrated cholesterol reductions of 11 percent to 32 percent with red yeast rice. American studies derived similar results:

- *American Journal of Clinical Nutrition:*

  In a double-blind, placebo-controlled study of 83 subjects, ages 34–78 with total cholesterol levels of 204–338 and LDL-C levels of 128–277, 1,200 mg of red yeast rice twice daily reduced LDL-C 22 percent on average, significantly better than placebo. No significant side effects occurred. The authors commented: "Red yeast rice significantly reduces total cholesterol, LDL cholesterol, and total triglyceride concentrations compared with placebo and provides a new, novel, food-based approach to lowering cholesterol in the general population."[5]

- *Nutrition:*

  In a small, placebo-controlled, double-blind study of AIDS patients with elevated cholesterol, 1,200 mg of red yeast rice twice-daily reduced LDL-C 32 percent on average. No side effects occurred.[6]

An additional benefit of red yeast rice is that, like prescription statins, it may reduce elevated C-reactive protein levels. Many alternative doctors prefer to treat elevated CRP with exercise, omega-3 oils, vitamin C, and/or vitamin E, which work sometimes. When these do not reduce CRP enough, a statin—a prescription statin or red yeast rice—may be useful.

Although red yeast rice is available over the counter, it should be used with medical supervision. Red yeast rice has been used in America for more than a decade, but at times it was difficult to obtain, so it hasn't been used extensively here. So far, its track record appears good. Reported side effects are few (headaches, stomach pain). Liver and kidney effects have not been seen in human studies,[7] but liver enzymes should be checked anyway. Like statin drugs, red yeast rice should not be used during pregnancy or with drugs contraindicated with statins.

Red yeast rice also provides an alternative for people who need but cannot afford prescription statins. Based on my own brief survey of pharmacies a few years ago, statins cost from $85 to $120 per month, whereas red yeast rice supplements cost only $20 to $30 per month. Red yeast rice is not FDA approved for reducing cholesterol or treating cardiovascular disease.

INTERMEDIATE-ACTING NIACIN

Niacin (nicotinic acid) is the rare therapy recommended by both mainstream and alternative doctors. Niacin was the first therapy proven to improve cholesterol levels. At doses much higher than the recommended daily allowance, niacin reduces total cholesterol and LDL-C, while raising HDL-C. Indeed, as a recent consumer health newsletter stated, "Niacin is the most potent pill you can take to raise your HDL ("good") cholesterol."[8] Niaspan, a prescription niacin preparation, can reduce LDL-C by 5 percent to 25 percent, triglycerides 20 percent to 50 percent, and increase HDL-C by 15 percent to 35 percent.[9]

Niacin is vitamin B_3, which is necessary for processing carbohydrates into energy or fat. Niacin also plays a role in the metabolism of cholesterol. Another form of vitamin B_3, niacinamide, has no effects on cholesterol metabolism. Niacin has favorable effects not only on cholesterol levels, but also on triglyceride and fibrinogen levels. It also reduces levels of small-particle LDL-C and lipoprotein A, which some doctors believe are more important risk indicators than a high LDL-C. Most important, niacin has been shown to reduce people's risk of heart attacks, including the risk of recurrent heart attacks in cardiac patients, and overall mortality.

As a result of niacin's beneficial effects on many cardiac risk factors, some physicians use it as a first-line therapy. Dr. Julian Whitaker states, "Niacin has been around for a long time as a cholesterol-lowering agent, and is the best single remedy for lowering LDL cholesterol and raising HDL."[10] Other doctors prefer using niacin as a second-line treatment or combined with other therapies. Because 25 percent to 50 percent of high-risk coronary patients do not reach their LDL-C goals even with the strongest statin doses,[11] niacin is often added.

Niacin can sometimes increase homocysteine levels. For a long time, niacin was thought to also increase blood glucose levels, but this does not seem to be the case for most people. However, if you take any form of niacin, your fasting serum glucose and homocysteine levels should be measured when your cholesterol levels are checked. Because niacin can raise uric acid levels or activate peptic ulcers, it is usually avoided in people with histories of gout or ulcers. Niacin is usually contraindicated if you have liver disease or consume substantial quantities of alcohol. All niacin products should be used cautiously with blood thinners.

Doctors generally do not recommend plain niacin because it is very short acting and frequently causes flushing, itching, headaches, and stomach pain. At the doses needed to benefit cholesterol levels, flushing can be intense and causes many people to quit treatment. These problems have led to the development of slowly absorbed, long-acting niacin products. However, some early sustained-release preparations caused liver toxicity, so intermediate-release (or "extended-release") niacin preparations, with better side-effect profiles, have become the preferred approach. These include prescription preparations such as Niaspan and over-the-counter inositol hexaniacinate.

Niaspan

Niaspan is the preferred niacin preparation among mainstream doctors, although some prescribe Niacor or generic equivalents. Niaspan is FDA approved and listed in the PDR, yet it does have some adverse effects. Flushing, warmth, redness, and itching occur less than with plain niacin, but still commonly occur. The manufacturer informs patients that taking aspirin or an anti-inflammatory drug such as ibuprofen thirty minutes before taking Niaspan may minimize flushing. Other adverse effects include headache, sweating, dizziness, nausea, heartburn, diarrhea, and palpitations.[12,13] Niaspan causes liver enzyme elevations in about 1 percent of patients and a reversible form of hepatitis can occur. Because Niaspan side effects are dose-related, as are most side effects of any niacin preparation, doctors usually initiate Niaspan therapy at 500 mg, then increase gradually to 1,000–2,000 mg/day. Women often respond to lower Niaspan doses than men. Liver enzyme levels should be checked regularly. Niaspan is a prescription drug and fairly expensive.

Advicor

Prescription Advicor contains 20 mg of Mevacor plus 500, 1,000, or 2,000 mg of Niaspan, thereby combining the cholesterol-lowering benefits of a statin and niacin. This combination is perhaps more convenient to use than two separate pills, but it does not allow you to start with a lower statin dose. Still, 20 mg of Mevacor is a modest amount and, combined with Niaspan, may provide the benefits that are preferable to high-dose statins.

Inositol Hexaniacinate (Hexanicotinate, Nicotinate)

Most alternative doctors I know prefer a different type of niacin derivative: inositol hexaniacinate. Inositol hexaniacinate is available over the counter and is much less expensive than Niaspan and Advicor. Inositol hexaniacinate appears to cause considerably fewer side effects than Niaspan, Advicor, or other standard, immediate- or extended-release types of niacin, as is shown by the following:

- *Alternative Medicine Review:*

  "The need for a safer approach to niacin supplementation has resulted in the investigation of niacin esters. One of the most widely studied of these is inositol hexaniacinate. In numerous trials it has been found virtually free of the side effects associated with conventional niacin therapy. Extensive research has found inositol hexaniacinate to be effective in the treatment of hyperlipidemia, Raynaud's disease and intermittent claudication."[14]

- *Nutrition Action Health Letter:*

  "The inositol hexaniacinate form of niacin has not been linked with the side effects associated with niacin supplementation. In a group of people being treated alternatively with niacin and inositol hexaniacinate for skin problems, niacin supplementation (50–100 mg per day) was associated with numerous side effects, including skin flushing, nausea, vomiting and agitation. In contrast, people taking inositol hexaniacinate experienced no complaints whatsoever, even at amounts two to five times higher than the previously used amounts of niacin."[8]

Dr. Jeffrey Baker, MD, an integrative family practitioner at the Immanuel Clinic in Springdale, AR, told me, "My first choice for reducing cholesterol is inositol hexaniacinate with a specific variety of antioxidants. I prescribe 600 mg twice daily. I believe the twice-daily approach is better than once-daily niacin therapies. I use inositol hexanicotinate a lot, and none of my patients have developed liver enzyme elevations."

In contrast, mainstream doctors stick with Niaspan and shy away from products not approved by the FDA because in the early 1980s, a popular over-the-counter sustained-release niacin product was associated with severe liver damage. But that was not inositol hexaniacinate, which despite widespread use has not shown any of these problems. Indeed, according to another in-depth review in the *Alternative Medicine Review,* "No adverse effects have been reported from the use of inositol hexaniacinate in dosages as high as four grams daily."[15] Studies dating back forty years indicate the effectiveness and safety of inositol hexaniacinate for a variety of cardiovascular disorders.

The actual mechanism of action of inositol hexaniacinate is not clear. Originally it was thought that when the body slowly metabolizes a molecule of inositol hexaniacinate over twelve hours, it releases six molecules of niacin. However, recent analyses suggest that little nicotinic acid is actually released in the blood of people taking inositol hexaniacinate. Whatever its exact mechanism, inositol hexaniacinate seems to have the same beneficial effects on cholesterol and other risk factor levels as standard niacin preparations.

Inositol hexaniacinate should be avoided in people with histories of liver disease. Liver enzyme levels should be checked when cholesterol levels are checked, especially if you are using doses above 2,000 mg/day. Inositol hexaniacinate is not FDA approved for treating lipid disorders or cardiovascular disease.

Which Type of Niacin Should You Use?

Good doctors disagree on this. Dr. Stephen Sinatra, who knows the mainstream and alternative methods for reducing cholesterol about as well as anyone, prefers Niaspan, usually at doses of 750 to 1,500 mg/day. But among his recommendations he adds: "Since therapeutic levels of niacin can cause an unpleasant flushing sensation and headache, gradually increase your dosage over several weeks or use the flush-free form of niacin, inositol hexaniacinate."[16]

Alternative physician Dr. Whitaker prefers inositol hexanicotinate, usually at 500 mg three times a day, but up to 1,000 mg three times a day (with close medical monitoring). Most integrative medicine practitioners I know prefer inositol hexaniacinate, while many mainstream doctors have been taught that inositol hexaniacinate does not work. My experience is that it does. My viewpoint is that if you have coronary or other atherosclerotic vascular disease or are otherwise at risk, it may be preferable to stick with the more proven product: Niaspan. But if you have moderate elevations of LDL-C or few risk factors, low HDL-C, or elevated levels of the other factors that niacin can reduce, why not try inositol hexaniacinate first? It is far less expensive and much less prone to vexing side effects. If it is not effective, you and your doctor can consider Niaspan or other interventions.

Whichever form of niacin is chosen, whether over-the-counter or prescription, I advise working closely with a healthcare practitioner. You will need to get blood tests anyway to know whether your cholesterol and/or other risk factors have been brought within target levels. Getting this right is too important to do blindly. Niacin preparations can affect glucose, uric acid, and liver enzyme levels, so these should be checked too.

POLICOSANOL (EXTRACT OF SUGAR CANE)

An intriguing characteristic of policosanol is its natural source. This makes policosanol an attractive alternative for a large number of patients who, although in dire need of lipid-lowering treatment, are reluctant to use chemically derived drugs and would gladly welcome a natural and efficient alternative.[17]

—AMERICAN HEART JOURNAL

Policosanol burst on the alternative medicine scene in early 2002. Its arrival was accompanied by an unusual amount of scientific evidence for a nutriceutical. In a series of well-designed double-blind, placebo-controlled studies conducted in Cuba, where policosanol was developed, the substance lowered total cholesterol and LDL-C, while raising HDL-C.

The following are some studies supporting the beneficial effects of policosanol:

- *American Heart Journal:*

   A review of twenty-one studies found that 10–20 mg of policosanol daily lowered total cholesterol 17 percent to 21 percent, LDL-C 21 percent to 29 percent, and raised HDL-C 8 percent to 15 percent, on average, with few side effects. The authors concluded: "Policosanol seems to be a very promising phytochemical alternative to classic lipid-lowering agents such as the statins."[17]

- *Current Therapeutics and Research:*

   In this double-blind, placebo-controlled study, 5 mg of policosanol daily reduced LDL-C 17.7 percent on average.[18]

- *Current Therapeutics and Research:*

   In a double-blind, placebo-controlled study, 5 mg of policosanol twice daily reduced LDL-C 21.5 percent on average.[19]

- *Current Therapeutics and Research:*

   In a double-blind, placebo-controlled study, 5 mg of policosanol twice-daily reduced LDL-C 21.2 percent, and 10 mg twice daily reduced LDL-C 30 percent on average.[20]

   Policosanol has also has been studied head-to-head against statins:

- *International Journal of Clinical Pharmacologic Research:*

   In this comparative double-blind trial, 10 mg of policosanol reduced LDL-C 19.3 percent on average; 10 mg of Pravachol reduced LDL-C by 15.6 percent.[21]

- *Current Therapeutics and Research:*

In this comparative, double-blind trial in elderly patients, 10 mg of policosanol reduced LDL-C 17.9 percent; 10 mg of Zocor reduced LDL-C 19.8 percent on average.[22]

- *Current Therapeutics and Research*:

  In a comparative, double-blind trial in patients with coronary risk factors, 10 mg of policosanol reduced LDL-C 32.4 percent; 20 mg of Mevacor reduced LDL-C 27.6 percent on average.[23]

These and many other studies are impressive, yet it is important to remember that policosanol is new. New chemicals—supplements as well as prescription drugs—should always be assessed carefully for their effectiveness. Moreover, "natural" doesn't automatically mean "safe." Because policosanol is relatively new to America, doctors in the U.S. have limited experience with it. Jacqueline Campbell, MD, of Jamaica, has been using policosanol for many years. "In my practice I have used policosanol. We get it directly from Cuba. I have found 10 mg to be very effective in lowering total cholesterol levels."

The starting dose of policosanol is 5 or 10 mg/day taken with dinner. A 20-mg dose is used for greater LDL-C reductions. Policosanol has no effect on triglycerides, and its effect on CRP is unknown. Policosanol is a mixture of alcohols (octacosanol, triacontanol, hexacosanol) isolated from purified sugar cane. It contains no sugar itself, however, so it can be used by diabetics. Policosanol appears to inhibit the production of cholesterol in the liver, but it does in a different way than statins and does not seem to inhibit coenzyme A or deplete coenzyme Q_{10}. Policosanol also reduces LDL-C oxidation (oxidation makes LDL-C more harmful to arteries), and it reduces platelet aggregation by inhibiting thromboxane B_2 and the smooth-muscle proliferation that may also play roles in the formation of atherosclerosis.[17] Studies show that policosanol improves cardiac function, reduces angina symptoms, and increases endurance in people with severe atherosclerosis in the legs.[24]

So far, policosanol appears to be quite safe. In long-term studies, side effects were infrequent and minor (headache, dizziness, nervousness, insomnia, sedation, stomach pain, increased urination),[24] but alternative doctors report few if any problems. It remains to be seen, however, whether policosanol is as good as advertised. Already there are reports that Americans do not derive as much benefit as the Cuban studies indicate. Some doctors report mixed results, with some patients responding well and other patients not responding. Other doctors say flatly that the policosanol available here does not work. Explanations for this include Americans' size or diets, or their more serious cholesterol problems, but the likely answer involves manufacturing practices. In America, most policosanol is derived from beets or beeswax instead of from sugar cane, which is the source of policosanol in Cuba. Because of the problems here, some American nutriceutical manufacturers are now producing policosanol from sugar cane with reportedly better and more consistent results in patients.

Policosanol may be worth trying if its benefits fit your needs and if you can obtain the sugar cane-based product. The cost is low: about $15 to $30 per month. Like red yeast rice, policosanol should be used with medical supervision. Policosanol is not FDA approved for reducing cholesterol or treating cardiovascular disease.

PLANT STEROLS

Plant sterols are recommended by the American Heart Association and the National Cholesterol Education Program Expert Panel as adjunct therapy to reduce LDL.[25]

—AMERICAN JOURNAL OF MANAGED CARE

Sterols are essential components of the cell membranes of animals and plants. In humans, cholesterol is the main sterol. Plants manufacture other sterols. When people eat plant sterols or their derivatives (plant stanols), these substances impair the absorption of cholesterol from the intestine. Studies have shown that 1.8 grams/day of plant sterols reduces LDL-C by 10 percent on average (range: 6 percent to 14 percent).[26,27] Higher doses provide little extra benefit. These LDL-C reductions are comparable to those obtained with prescription drugs that block cholesterol absorption, such as cholestyramine, Welchol, and Zetia, and plant sterols are less expensive and less side effect-prone.

Plant sterols can be used with other cholesterol-lowering therapies. An article in the *Medical Journal of Australia* stated that "phytosterol-containing foods are valuable additions to other cholesterol-lowering treatments, including statins."[28] The *Journal of Nutrition* concurred: "It has been demonstrated that foods enriched with plant sterols and stanols are effective in various population groups, and in combination with cholesterol-lowering diets or drugs."[29] This is why both the National Institutes of Health and the U.S. Food and Drug Administration support the use of plant sterols for lowering cholesterol and reducing the risk of heart disease.

Plant sterols are present in small amounts in vegetable oils, seeds, nuts, and some vegetables and fruits. Margarines enriched with plant sterols are available today, but these should be avoided if they contain trans fats. You can buy supplements with plant sterols and stanols in health food stores. Plant sterols appear to cause few side effects in humans. There is some evidence that they may block the absorption of fat-soluble vitamins, especially carotene, which can be offset by an extra portion of an orange or yellow vegetable or fruit. The long-term effects of plant sterols are not known.

FIBER

There are two types of fiber: soluble and insoluble. Soluble fiber breaks down within the digestive tract and is absorbed into the body, while insoluble fiber passes through the intestines essentially unchanged. Soluble fiber can lower blood cholesterol and triglyceride levels. Both types of fiber can reduce hypertension and blood glucose levels.[30] Both types of fibers have been shown to reduce the risk of heart disease, and insoluble fiber is associated with reduced risks of diverticulitis, and colon and breast cancer.

Dietary fiber comes from the thick cell walls of plants. Whole grains are good sources of insoluble fiber. Both types of fiber can be obtained from oats, barley, beans, vegetables, legumes, and whole fruit. Unfortunately, the typical western diet is low in fiber content, providing about 10 grams/day of fiber. Our ancestors got 40 to 60 grams of fiber a day from their unprocessed foods. The FDA, the National Academy of Sciences, and the American Cancer Society recommend 25 to 35 grams of fiber per day.

Dr. Andrew Weil recommends dietary fiber among his cardiovascular health strategies: "Soluble fiber has a powerful cholesterol-lowering effect. The best sources of soluble fiber are beans and lentils, apples, citrus fruits, oats, barley, peas, carrots."[31] Packaged forms of soluble fiber include psyllium and pectin. The use of psyllium has been shown to allow statin patients to use lower statin doses. Chitosan, a new form of fiber derived from shellfish, has also produced some very good initial results.

GUGGULIPID (GUGGUL, GUGUL)

Guggulipid is an extract of Gum guggul, a natural Ayurvedic medicine used in India for centuries. Guggulipid not only reduces cholesterol, but also acts as an antioxidant and reduces platelet aggregation. According to *The People's Pharmacy*, guggulipid is approved in India for lowering cholesterol and preventing heart disease. Guggulipid's active ingredient is guggulsterone. The mechanism of action is not clear, but guggulipid appears to block LDL-C production or transport, and may block the absorption of cholesterol from the intestine. Another explanation is that guggulipid facilitates the production of bile acids, thereby enhancing the removal of cholesterol from the body. Guggulipid does not appear to deplete coenzyme Q_{10}.

The standard dose of guggulipid is 250 or 500 mg twice daily with meals; 500 mg three times a day is also used. Or 25 mg of guggulsterone is used three times a day with meals. Side effects include nausea, gas, and bloating.

Most studies of guggulipid have been conducted in India:

- *Cardiovascular Drugs and Therapeutics:*
  In this double-blind, placebo-controlled study of 50 mg of guggulsterone twice daily in thirty-one patients, guggulipid reduced total cholesterol by 11.7 percent, LDL-C 12.5 percent, triglycerides 12 percent.[32]

- *Journal of the Association of Physicians of India:*
  A twelve-week open trial involving 205 patients. 500 mg of guggulipid three times a day reduced total cholesterol 23.6 percent and triglycerides 22.6 percent on average. Only one patient reported side effects (stomach pain). In a second double-blind phase, 125 patients taking guggulipid were compared with 108 patients taking the prescription drug clofibrate. Guggulipid reduced total cholesterol 11 percent and triglycerides 16.8 percent on average. Clofibrate reduced total cholesterol 10 percent and triglycerides 21.6 percent.[33]

Most striking about the latter study is the difference in cholesterol reduction—24 percent versus 11 percent—achieved in the study's two phases. Interestingly, doctors tell me the same thing. Some doctors report excellent results with guggulipid, while others do not. Dr. Baker told me, "I haven't seen impressive results. Other alternative methods work better." Yet a review in the *American Family Physician* concluded that preliminary results with guggulipid are promising and toxicities appear to be few.[4] The operative word was "preliminary," because very few studies had been done. This changed in 2003 with the publication of the first major study in western patients taking guggulipid.

In this double-blind study, 103 patients received 1,000 or 2,000 mg of guggulipid or a placebo three times a day. The results: guggulipid actually raised LDL-C levels slightly and had no beneficial effect on total cholesterol, triglycerides, or HDL-C. Moreover, six people developed rashes with guggulipid compared to none with placebo.[34] When asked about the results, Dr. Philippe O. Szapary, who led the study, said, "The bottom line is, if you are trying to lower your [cholesterol], don't use guggulipid. There are plenty of proven safe and effective therapies on the market. We need to spend time and money investigating these products."[35] That's true, but no supplement manufacturer has the deep pockets of the drug companies, so studies on non-drug alternatives are sporadic.

This study made health-page headlines, and the articles were distinctly negative about guggulipid. Yet, a close reading of the published study revealed that high-dose guggulipid reduced median levels of CRP by 25 percent, which I confirmed in correspondence with Dr. Szapary.[36] This is a significant and important finding, especially because CRP went up 30 percent in the placebo group. Low-dose guggulipid had no effect on CRP. Because more and more doctors believe that the inflammation reflected by CRP measurements is as important a risk factor as LDL-C levels, the impact of high-dose guggulipid on CRP may explain its long use in Ayurvedic medicine.

Where does this leave guggulipid as a treatment for atherosclerosis? On uncertain ground. Guggulipid may have an important role in reducing CRP, and in some patients, it may have beneficial effects on cholesterol levels. Because of the uncertainty, guggulipid should be used with medical monitoring of cholesterol and CRP levels. Guggulipid is not FDA approved for reducing cholesterol or CRP, or for treating cardiovascular disease.

GARLIC

Garlic is said to reduce LDL-C and triglyceride levels, and to prevent the harmful oxidation of LDL-C. However, studies on garlic's cholesterol-lowering abilities are mixed. An earlier review of garlic studies showed that garlic reduced total cholesterol by 12 percent.[37] However, in recent studies, garlic's effects have been less impressive. A study using two different doses of a garlic supplement showed no effect with the lower dose and a 6.1 percent reduction in total cholesterol with the higher dose.[38] A study of Kyolic garlic showed a modest 4 percent reduction in LDL-C; more impressive was its reduction of systolic blood pressure by 5.5 percent.[39]

A comprehensive review of garlic studies in the *Annals of Internal Medicine* found that garlic reduced cholesterol levels by 7 percent on average. The authors concluded: "The available data suggest that garlic is superior to placebo in reducing total cholesterol levels. However, the size of the effect is modest." They concluded that using garlic to reduce cholesterol levels was "questionable."[40] An article in the *American Family Physician* went further: "Despite the many early promising studies and meta-analyses evaluating garlic's effect as a lipid-lowering agent, more recent, rigorous studies have failed to substantiate these benefits. There is no current role for garlic as an antihyperlipidemic agent."[4]

Garlic's effects on cholesterol levels and blood pressure may be modest on average, but some people attest to getting good results. Dr. Whitaker states, "Garlic promotes an optimum ratio of LDL-to-HDL cholesterol and promotes elastic artery walls."[41] He recommends garlic in combination with guggulipid, flax, niacin, and B-vitamins. Dr. Weil recommends fresh garlic: "Garlic has been shown to lower both cholesterol levels and blood pressure—and it tastes wonderful, too. Use one or two lightly cooked cloves a day."[31]

Garlic's safety is established, and its cost is low. Even with modest results, garlic can serve as an adjunct to other methods of reducing cholesterol, allowing you to use lower doses of cholesterol-lowering drugs or other supplements. Garlic is not FDA approved for reducing cholesterol or treating cardiovascular disease. Garlic can cause mild inhibition of platelets, so you should discontinue using it at least one week before having surgery.

SOY

The FDA has approved this health claim:

> 25 grams of soy protein a day, as part of a diet low in saturated fat and cholesterol, may reduce the risk of heart disease.[42]

Indeed, studies dating back as far as 1941 have demonstrated soy's beneficial effects on cholesterol levels. Studies show that soy protein reduces total cholesterol about 9 percent, LDL-C 13 percent, and triglycerides 10 percent, on average.[4,43,44] But soy's effect on these factors is variable: some people obtain substantial cholesterol reductions, others do not. New evidence suggests that soy may also favorably influence the size of LDL-C particles.[45]

Getting 25 grams of soy protein daily is not easy. Two ounces of tofu contain 8.5 grams of soy protein, and there are just so many soy burgers and hot dogs you can eat. Soy milk, soy flour, soy puddings, and supplements are other ways of getting soy.

However, some experts have expressed concern about using soy in large quantities. Dr. Sherry Rogers, a leading voice in alternative medicine, does not recommend soy because of its estrogenic effects. Drs. Daniel Shee-han and Daniel Doerge, FDA experts on soy, argued against approving the soy health statement because of soy's effects on estrogen-sensitive tissues and the thyroid.[46] Joseph Mercola, MD, who produces one of the most popular health websites in the world (*www.mercola.com*), is not fond of soy: "Soy is not the health food that it's made out to be. I regularly see women who have thyroid problems as a result of consuming soy."[47]

Other doctors strongly disagree and recommend moderate amounts of soy and believe it can play a role in heart health and longevity. Dr. Whitaker states, "Soybeans are an excellent source of high-quality protein, fiber, sterols, and specialized phytonutrients known as isoflavones, powerful antioxidants that protect the arteries, lower cholesterol, discourage LDL-C oxidation, and help prevent the formation of potentially dangerous blood clots." Whitaker acknowledges that some doctors disagree, but adds, "I've looked at this issue from every angle, and I remain convinced that the good outweighs the bad."[48] He recommends that people eat soy several times a week.

An analysis in *Consumer Reports* concluded: "A large body of evidence shows that soy can be good for most people. Soy protein, which can help lower cholesterol and reduce the risk of heart attack, contains the nine essential amino acids found in animal protein, but it is much lower in saturated fat and has no cholesterol." Noting the FDA's approval of soy and that 25 mg/day of soy protein can lower total cholesterol by 5 percent to 10 percent, the magazine added "such reductions should produce a 10 percent to 30 percent drop in heart attack risk."[49]

It would be comforting if this were the last word, but around the same time, the *Los Angeles Times* stated "soy has been losing luster for years." The emerging research on soy has not upheld the FDA's health claim, according to Alice Lichtenstein, a professor of nutrition science at Tufts University. Soy, she stated, has "very little effect" on lowering LDL-C.[50] Yet Dr. Steven Pratt, in his bestseller *Superfoods*, lists soy as one of the top fourteen foods you can eat. Dr. Pratt specifically mentions soy's ability to reduce cholesterol.[51]

Clearly, the final chapter on soy remains to be written. In the meantime, you can try soy products and see whether they help reduce your total cholesterol and LDL-C levels. It may be that soy is helpful for some but not others. If you get a 5 percent to 10 percent reduction from soy, and you combine this with other nutritional and other lifestyle efforts, you will be doing a lot to maintain cardiovascular health.

PROMISING NEW NATURAL THERAPIES

The two most promising new natural therapies I have seen are tocotrienols and pantethine. Tocotrienols are similar in structure to vitamin E (tocopherols). Early evidence shoes that tocotrienols can reduce total cholesterol, LDL-C, and triglyceride levels. Tocotrienols are especially effective when combined with a heart-healthy diet. Several manufacturers are offering balanced formulas containing tocotrienols and two forms of vitamin E, alpha and gamma.

Pantethine is a derivative of vitamin B_5 (pantothenic acid). Early evidence indicates that pantethine can reduce total cholesterol, LDL-C, and triglyceride levels, and raise HDL-C. Pantethine also possesses anti-inflammatory and antioxidant qualities.

As this chapter demonstrates, there are many natural therapies that can be used with or instead of statins. Many of these therapies are supported by solid science and the positive experiences of patients. Although these therapies are available without a prescription, I advise people to work with a knowledgeable healthcare provider in deciding among the many choices and doses of natural therapies and in monitoring their effects on cholesterol and CRP levels.

9

Essential Nutrients
for Cardiovascular Health

The precision-prescribing method considers not only the disease at hand, but all of the factors that might have prevented the disease and the factors that can help reduce its severity or progression. Thus, it is not enough to simply select a pill to lower cholesterol. Optimal health means considering methods that can improve overall functioning of the heart and blood vessels. Statins have their benefits, but they do not restore health to an unhealthy vascular system or improve deficiencies of key nutrients in cells.

People usually think of omega-3 oils, coenzyme Q_{10}, folic acid, and magnesium as supplements, but they aren't. They are nutrients. They are substances that are requisite parts of our physiology, needed by human cells and structures just like amino acids, vitamin C, and calcium, and necessary for proper body functioning. Yet most people are severely deficient in omega-3 oils and magnesium, and coenzyme Q_{10} and folic acid are particularly important for cardiovascular health, yet they are routinely ignored in mainstream medicine today.

OMEGA-3 FATTY ACIDS (FISH OILS, ESSENTIAL FATTY ACIDS)

Failure to eat enough essential fatty acids is a cause of hardening of the arteries, abnormal clot formation, coronary heart disease, high cholesterol, and high blood pressure.[1]

—EDWARD SIGUEL, MD, PHD

Omega-3 fatty acids (EPA and DHA) may be as important as any of the pharmaceuticals and nutriceuticals discussed in this book. The human

119

body cannot make all of the kinds of fats it requires. Some fats are *essential*: they must be obtained from foods. These essential oils are linolenic and linoleic, which provide omega-3 and omega-6 fatty acids, respectively. Omega-3 and omega-6 fatty acids serve many vital functions in the body, and one of their foremost functions is to maintain cardiovascular health. Together, omega-3 and omega-6 fatty acids reduce LDL-C and raise HDL-C. Higher doses of omega-3 oils also reduce triglyceride levels. But it is not that simple, because in modern countries today, most people get too many omega-6 oils from the corn, soy, safflower, sunflower, peanut, and cottonseed oils that are used so widely in packaged foods, salad dressings, and fast foods. Worse, very few people get enough omega-3 fatty oils, which are plentiful only in fatty fish (sardines, ocean salmon, swordfish, and tuna that is not nonfat) and flaxseeds, and getting enough omega-3 oils is fundamental to maintaining cardiovascular health.

The importance of omega-3 oils did not become well known until the late 1990s, and a lot of people still haven't gotten the word. Scientists did not know about omega-3 oils until the late 1970s, when studies showed that Eskimos, despite fat-laden diets, had substantially fewer heart attacks than people in industrialized societies. These findings defied the accepted wisdom that excess fat in the diet causes atherosclerosis and heart disease. The observation that the fat from fish might be beneficial launched a new area of research, as described in the *Mayo Clinic Proceedings:*

> These observations generated more than 4,500 studies to explore this and other effects of omega-3 fatty acids on human metabolism and health. From epidemiology to cell culture and animal studies to randomized controlled trials, the cardioprotective effects of omega-3 fatty acids are becoming recognized.[2]

Such recognition has come slowly. It was not until a large, placebo-controlled Italian study, known as the GISSI study, was published in *Lancet* in 1999 that mainstream medicine began to take serious notice. In this study, more than 11,000 people with recent heart attacks were given 1 gram/day of omega-3 oils or placebo for three and a half years. Over just three and a half years, the omega-3 group had significantly fewer heart attacks and strokes, cardiac death was reduced 45 percent, and death from all causes was reduced 20 percent.[3] Today, it is widely accepted that omega-3 fatty acids reduce heart attacks, strokes, and deaths from heart disease, as well as the overall incidence of death from all causes.

Evidence-Based Information on Benefits of Omega-3 Fatty Acids

Here is a small sample of the many articles in the medical literature about the benefits of omega-3 fatty acids.

■ *European Heart Journal:* "Sudden cardiac death is very common . . . and accounts for about 50 percent of cardiovascular mortality in developed countries . . . . Clinical and epidemiological studies, and randomized trials, clearly demonstrated that omega-3 polyunsaturated fatty acids reduce the risk of sudden cardiac death. Their clinical use is now encouraged."[4]

■ *New England Journal of Medicine:* "The omega-3 fatty acids found in fish are strongly associated with a reduced risk of sudden death among men without evidence of prior cardiovascular disease." Compared with men with the lowest levels of omega-3 fatty acids, the men in this study with the highest levels of omega-3s "had an 81 percent lower risk of sudden death."[5]

■ *JAMA:* "Among women, higher consumption of fish and omega-3 fatty acids is associated with a lower risk of coronary heart disease, particularly coronary heart disease deaths . . . . In our study, omega-3 fatty acid intake and fish consumption were associated with a significantly lower risk of coronary heart disease."[6]

■ *Circulation:* "A growing consensus for a direct relationship between increased intake of omega-3 fatty acids either from dietary sources or as a pharmacological supplementation and decreasing risk of coronary heart disease has become apparent over the years." In this study: "Patients allocated to omega-3 fatty acids treatment had a significantly lower mortality even after only 3 months of treatment."[7]

■ *Public Health and Nutrition:* "For decades it has been postulated that the main environmental factor for coronary heart disease was the intake of saturated fatty acids. Nevertheless, confirmation of the role of saturated fatty acids in coronary heart disease through intervention trials has been disappointing. It was only when the diet was enriched with omega-3 fatty acids that coronary heart disease was significantly prevented, especially cardiac death."[8]

We also know that omega-3 oils are a critical factor in keeping blood vessels functioning properly and in preventing cardiac arrhythmias when heart attacks occur. For many people, the first symptom of heart disease is a heart attack. Each year, 250,000 people die from sudden cardiac death,

ˌeart attacks that are not in themselves lethal, but which trig-
ˌs that are. Multiple studies have now proven that omega-3 oils
ˌisk of sudden cardiac death by an astounding 40 percent to 80
peˌ ˌee the inset on page 121).[4-9] "The higher your blood level of
omega-ˌ, the lower your risk" of sudden cardiac death, says Dr. Christine
M. Albert, the chief of cardiology at Massachusetts General Hospital and the
lead author of a major study on this issue.[5]

Despite these proven benefits, mainstream doctors often fail to suggest
omega-3 oils to patients. And despite headlines in the mainstream media
about studies proving the benefits of omega-3 oils, this issue is not mentioned when famous people die suddenly from heart attacks. In the sports
world in 2002 and 2003, lethal heart attacks struck Johnny Unitas (football),
32-year-old Darryl Kile (baseball), and Dave DeBusschere (basketball)—all
former all-stars. Yet, in the stories about these legends' deaths, not a question was asked about their diets or their intakes of fish or omega-3 oils. Not
a word was written that these deaths might have been preventable. So what
I call the *Unitas-Kile-DeBusschere Syndrome*—sudden cardiac death—continues to go unrecognized and uncorrected in our society. This is unfortunate
because most westerners are deficient in omega-3 oils, and eating fatty fish
once weekly or taking two to three fish oil capsules a day is not only recommended by the Expert U.S. Panel and the British Nutrition Foundation,
but also easy and inexpensive.

Because they are essential nutrients, omega-3 oils have many other benefits. Omega-3 oils improve the functioning of the endothelium lining the
insides of arteries. Omega-3 oils have anti-inflammatory effects that may be
helpful in reducing C-reactive protein levels and preventing artery damage
and atherosclerosis. Studies have shown that men with high levels of arterial inflammation are far more likely to have heart attacks and strokes than
men with low levels of inflammation.[10, 11] Omega-3 oils are the body's natural anti-inflammatory substances. They also inhibit the platelet clumping
and the clotting that contributes to coronary disease and strokes. These
properties are reasons why the American Heart Association recommends at
least two servings of fish a week.[12]

Due to their anti-inflammatory effect, high doses of omega-3 oils have
proven beneficial in studies of autoimmune disorders such as rheumatoid
arthritis and Crohn's disease, so omega-3s should also help reduce CRP. Yet
studies of omega-3 oils for CRP have been equivocal, probably because the
doses studied were inadequate. Authorities recommend 2 to 3 grams of fish
oil daily to reduce cardiac arrhythmias, but inflammatory disorders like

rheumatoid arthritis or lupus require 6 to 12 grams per day. These higher doses may also be necessary for reducing elevated CRP. The studies on omega-3 oils for CRP may also have been too brief. Correcting deficiencies of omega-3 oils takes time. Restoring the balance of essential oils in all of your 50 trillion cells cannot be done overnight. This usually takes four to six months and also requires a reduction in pro-inflammatory omega-6 oils.

Omega-3 oils are something on which mainstream and alternative doctors agree. Dr. Andrew Weil says, "The omega-3 fatty acids in fish and fish oil supplements have been shown to be an effective preventive strategy against heart disease. They can lower triglyceride levels, increase HDL-C, help minimize inflammation and blood clotting, and keep blood vessels healthy."[13] Dr. Stephen Sinatra adds, "The EPA contained in fish oil is a terrific anti-inflammatory agent. And the DHA in fish oil has been shown to help minimize asthma and arthritis, along with inflammation caused by cancer."[14]

Indeed, omega-3 oils also may help prevent cancer of the breast, colon, and prostate. Omega-3 oils improve glucose metabolism, reduce insulin reactivity, and reduce blood pressure. Omega-3 oils reduce triglyceride levels, but have variable effects on LDL-C. But when taken with a small amount of gamma-linoleic acid (GLA), an omega-6 fatty acid, LDL-C levels are reduced.

How can you get more omega-3 oils? Some experts recommend eating fatty fish once or twice a week to obtain the heart benefits, but others discourage this because of toxins that accumulate in the fat of these fish. The FDA already warns pregnant women against eating too much fish because of the effects of mercury on developing children, and that was before 2003, when the FDA lowered its safety standard for mercury in humans to one-quarter its previous amount. High levels of mercury have also been associated with infertility.[15] Joseph Mercola, MD, recommends avoiding most fish. "Some fish have less mercury than others, but nearly all fish are contaminated with mercury. I have done thousands of hair mineral analyses on patients . . . [and] patients who don't eat any fish are the only ones who have immeasurable levels of mercury in their hair. Anyone eating fish has mercury in their system, and it is nearly always in direct proportion to the frequency of their fish consumption." Exceptions are sardines and anchovies, which have little mercury, probably because they haven't been in the ocean long enough to accumulate a lot in their tissues.[16] Other experts disagree with Dr. Mercola's perspective and contend that a moderate intake of fish is safe and beneficial.

Do the fish you eat actually contain omega-3 oils? Much of the salmon offered at markets today is farmed. These fish receive feeds that are not like the natural plankton eaten by wild fish and do not stimulate the production of as much omega-3 oils. Moreover, a recent report showed higher levels of toxins in farmed fish. So if you want to eat fish in order to obtain omega-3 oils, choose wild ocean fish.

Early man had no difficulty getting enough omega-3 oils. His diet relied on free ranging animals, which manufactured omega-3 oils naturally from the grasses they ate. Modern man gets meat from animals raised on grains, which aren't their natural foods and don't allow their bodies to produce much omega-3 oil. This is why alternative doctors like Dr. Mercola now recommend range-raised beef whose main feed is grass.

The easiest and most reliable way of getting enough omega-3 oils is from fish oil capsules. Quality is the key here, and high-quality capsules have had the omega-3 oils cleaned and detoxified of metals, pesticides, and other toxins. Then the oils are combined with a little vitamin E to maintain freshness. High-quality fish oil capsules should have no odor or fishy taste. A gram of fish oil usually provides 300 mg of omega-3 oils (EPA and DHA). Some companies are making more potent capsules containing 500 mg of omega-3 oils, meaning fewer capsules and fewer calories. Others are marketing potent capsules containing only DHA, but I prefer capsules with a balance of EPA and DHA.

In order to maximize the anti-inflammatory effects of omega-3 oils, you may have to reduce your intake of pro-inflammatory omega-6 oils. The idea of limiting omega-6 oils is controversial. Some experts disagree with limiting omega-6 oils, but Dr. Artemis Simopoulos, who for decades has been the foremost researcher and educator about omega-3 oils, recommends limiting omega-6s. Studies of autoimmune diseases also suggest that limiting omega-6 oils while increasing omega-3s is necessary for reducing inflammation.

The fact is, most people are already saturated with omega-6 oils. Healthy diets should provide a ratio of omega-6/omega-3 oils of 2:1 or 1:1, but western diets are so imbalanced toward omega-6 oils, the ratio is closer to 17:1. People are supposed to get about 1 gram of omega-3 oils daily, but the average intake is about 0.1–0.2 grams/day. This dietary imbalance of too much pro-inflammatory omega-6 and too little anti-inflammatory omega-3 may explain why inflammatory diseases and inflammation of the arteries are so widespread today. To correct the balance, you need an omega-6/omega-3 intake that approaches 1:1.

Which oils can you use? Olive oil is preferred. Scores of studies of people eating Mediterranean diets rich in olive oil demonstrate much lower incidences of cardiovascular disease and much greater longevity. Olive oil contains many healthful constituents and is loaded with antioxidants. When olive oil can't be used, I prefer canola oil, which does contain some omega-6 fatty acids but also contains omega-3s. Dr. Mercola recommends coconut oil for cooking because, despite its high saturated fat content, it does not break down when subjected to intense heat. And don't forget to also include some omega-6 oils, because they are essential oils, too.

Do omega-3 oils have a downside? Large amounts of fish oils are said to increase bleeding tendencies, although reports of this are few, and none of the mainstream or alternative doctors I know who use fish oils have seen any problems. Nevertheless, fish oils should be used carefully with aspirin and are contraindicated with blood thinners. In fact, some people take fish oils instead of aspirin to prevent heart disease. While doctors strongly recommend daily low-dose aspirin for people with heart disease, aspirin is not recommended for others. Many people use aspirin anyway, but aspirin has its own risks such as gastric bleeding or increased bleeding from trauma such as automobile accidents. Fish oils may offer a safer alternative. High doses of omega-3 oils should be taken with a doctor's supervision. If you are taking high doses of fish oil supplements, you should have your doctor check your cellular levels of omega-3 and omega-6 fatty acids with your other annual laboratory tests. Fish oil supplements are not FDA approved for reducing cholesterol or treating cardiovascular disease.

COENZYME Q_{10}

Coenzyme Q_{10} is a powerful antioxidant that enhances energy production in the mitochondria of cells, inhibits the oxidation of LDL-C, and has shown benefit in coronary disease, arrhythmias, congestive heart failure, and hypertension. Coenzyme Q_{10}'s benefits have been demonstrated in dozens of studies. "Coenzyme Q_{10}—CoQ_{10}—the nutrient I can't imagine practicing medicine without," states Dr. Sinatra. "CoQ_{10} supports healthy HDL and prevents the excess oxidation of LDL." Dr. Sinatra recommends 45 to 90 mg of softgel CoQ_{10} daily, but much higher doses for people with congestive heart failure. He also recommends 30 to 90 mg per day of CoQ_{10} for women over 30, because women are more vulnerable than men to CoQ_{10} deficiency.[11]

Dr. Julian Whitaker concurs: "Every patient I treat who has heart disease is immediately placed on CoQ_{10}. CoQ_{10} deficiencies and heart failure go hand in hand, and patients with the lowest levels generally have the most severe disease."[176] Dr. Whitaker recounts cases in which CoQ_{10} produced remarkable improvement in people with severe, end-stage congestive heart failure. As discussed in Chapter 4, Dr. Whitaker has petitioned the FDA to require a warning in statin package inserts about the importance of taking coenzyme Q_{10} with statins.

Coenzyme Q_{10} is another extensively studied nutrient that mainstream doctors are just now learning about, but alternative doctors have been recommending for years. Many alternative doctors believe that the muscle pain and fatigue accompanying statin therapy is caused by statins blocking the body's production of CoQ_{10}, and they attest that CoQ_{10} reduces or eliminates these side effects. In fact, some alternative doctors prescribe statins, but when they do, they also recommend CoQ_{10}.

CoQ_{10} is not FDA approved for reducing cholesterol or treating cardiovascular disease.

FOLIC ACID

You can't say, "Well, I'll take folic acid and eat whatever I want." But I do recommend folic acid for all of my patients.[18]

—CRAIG SCOTT, MD

In the rush to embrace C-reactive protein as the explanation for why 50 percent of heart attacks occur in people with normal cholesterol levels, folic acid should not be forgotten. Folic acid does not reduce cholesterol, but it does reduce homocysteine, which at elevated levels is directly linked to coronary artery disease. Elevated homocysteine is also linked to an increased incidence of congestive heart failure.[19] The large National Health and Nutrition Examination Survey (NHANES I) found that low folic acid intakes were associated with higher rates of strokes and other cardiovascular disorders.[20] Yet doctors have long overlooked and underutilized folic acid for reducing people's cardiovascular risk. Elevated homocysteine levels have also been linked to impaired cognitive functioning and Parkinson's and Alzheimer's diseases in the elderly, pregnancy complications, birth defects, increased death rates in diabetics, and possibly cancer. As mentioned in Chapter 2, elevated homocysteine levels develop in people who are unable to fully metabolize the amino acid methionine, which is abundant in meat. Reducing the intake of animal protein can lower homocysteine levels. Folic acid, with vitamin B_{12} and low doses of vitamin B_6, is effective in facilitating the metabolism of methionine, thereby reducing homocysteine levels.

How much folic acid do you need? The U.S. recommended daily allowance is 400 micrograms/day (0.4 milligrams/day). However, for people with atherosclerosis, a study in the *American Journal of Hypertension* found that 2.5 mg/day of folic acid, 0.25 mg B_{12}, plus 25 mg of B_6 reversed artery clogging.[21] Another study found that older people need at least 1 mg/day of folic acid for its cardiovascular benefits.[22] Some people may need much larger doses. "About 30% of my patients with elevated homocysteine don't use folic acid very efficiently," states Dr. Neil Hirschenbein of La Jolla, CA. "Some people need 10 or even 20 mg of folic acid a day."[23]

Some people cannot metabolize folic acid to its active form in their cells. If this is the case, you can purchase the active form, L-5-MTHF (L-5-methyl tetrahydrofolate), from some supplement companies. Trimethylglycine (TMG) can also be used to reduce homocysteine levels.

Although most doctors know that elevated homocysteine can damage blood vessels and cause narrowing of arteries, relatively few doctors order homocysteine level tests for their patients. Ask your doctor about including a homocysteine level in your next blood study. Normal homocysteine levels are usually defined as up to 20 micromoles per liter (µmol/L) of plasma, but some experts believe that a level above 9 is too high.[21] "Our own laboratory still defines normal as below 20 micromoles," Dr. Mimi Guarneri, cardiologist and medical director of the Scripps Clinic Center for Integrative Medicine, stated at a recent conference. "But I believe normal homocysteine levels are less than 9."

Some alternative doctors advise levels a bit lower: 7 or below. Hopefully, mainstream medicine and mainstream laboratories will get the word soon, because new studies suggest that for each 5 µmol/L elevation in homocysteine levels, cardiovascular risk increases by 60 percent in men and 80 percent in women.[24]

MAGNESIUM

Magnesium does not lower cholesterol or CRP, but it is so important for cardiac and vascular health, it must be mentioned.

The medical literature is filled with hundreds upon hundreds of studies such as these regarding magnesium's beneficial effects:

- *U.S. National Institutes of Health:*
  "Magnesium deficiency can cause metabolic changes that may contribute to heart attacks and strokes. Population surveys have associated higher

blood levels of magnesium with lower risk of coronary heart disease . . . and of stroke."[25]

■ *Medicinski Pregled [Medical Review (Croatia)]*

"It has been accepted by authors all over the world that the role of magnesium is of great importance in the prevention and treatment of cardiac patients."[26]

■ *USA Weekend:*

"Minus magnesium, hearts beat irregularly; arteries stiffen, constrict and clog; blood pressure rises; blood tends to clot; muscles spasm; insulin grows weaker and blood sugar jumps; bones lose strength; and pain signals intensify."[27]

■ *African Journal of Medicine and Medical Science:*

"Congestive heart failure is associated with electrolyte imbalance including magnesium deficit, which may increase myocardial electrical instability, risk of arrhythmias, and sudden death."[28]

There is an astonishing amount of scientific articles on magnesium. Magnesium's importance for general and cardiovascular health is indisputable. "Magnesium has a well-deserved reputation as the number 1 cardiovascular disease prevention mineral," states Jonathan Wright, MD, an early pioneer of the alternative medicine movement.[29] Dr. Sinatra adds, "Magnesium, the unsung hero of heart health, can be life-saving, especially for those who have suffered a heart attack or are at high risk; are prone to ventricular arrhythmias; are planning open-heart surgery; have congestive heart failure or cardiomyopathy; have high blood pressure; or are on long-term diuretics."[30] As many as 75 percent of people in western societies are magnesium deficient, yet most mainstream doctors do not know about it, and standard magnesium tests are not accurate enough to show even major deficiencies. Most people do not get anywhere near the RDA of 320 to 400 mg of magnesium in their diets, and some experts believe that the RDA is too low. Alternative doctors often recommend 500 to 1,000 mg/day.

The best known magnesium supplements are inexpensive, inorganic salts such as magnesium oxide that are poorly absorbed, causing gas or diarrhea. However, getting enough magnesium is essential for treating many cardiovascular conditions, including hypertension, Raynaud's phenomenon, and migraines. In fact, although magnesium is rarely used by mainstream doctors for treating office patients, it is frequently used in urgent care centers because of its proven ability to relax blood vessels and to reduce excitability of heart and brain cells. Intravenous magnesium is used in cardiac care units for cardiac arrhythmias and on obstetrical floors for eclampsia, which causes acute hypertension and seizures in pregnant women.

Magnesium was the key to my overcoming a very rare, severe vascular disease known as erythromelalgia. After trying scores of drugs, medical procedures, and alternative methods that did not work, I finally got improvement with prescription calcium channel blockers. But even at modest doses, I could not handle their side effects and found, to my own edification, that magnesium worked better with no side effects. I also learned that magnesium is needed to balance calcium in blood vessels and muscles, thereby reducing muscle tension and nerve excitability. After I had been disabled for years, magnesium gradually got me into a remission that has lasted several years. As the Chairman of the Medical Advisory Committee of The Erythromelalgia Association, I have recommended magnesium to scores of people and have learned that magnesium helps some but not others. This is not surprising because of the great variability in response seen with most therapies for vascular diseases such as hypertension and migraines. The fact that magnesium helps about 50 percent—people who had not responded to dozens of other treatments—is pretty good, better and safer and far less expensive than many highly touted drugs.

I want to underscore the importance of magnesium in helping people prevent hypertension, which is the single greatest contributor to cardiovascular disease. How serious is this wear and tear caused by hypertension? *Conn's Current Therapy,* a leading medical reference, describes it this way:

A 35-year-old man with an arterial pressure of 130/90 will die 4 years earlier than another 35-year-old man with the same medical background but with normal pressure. If his pressure is 140/90, he will die 9 years earlier, and if it's 150/100, he will die 17 years earlier.[31]

Although this book focuses on maintaining cardiovascular health by reducing cholesterol, CRP, homocysteine, and other atherosclerosis-causing factors, hypertension is a more serious and more certain risk factor for vascular damage, heart attacks, and strokes than any of them. If you have hypertension and high cholesterol or high CRP and must treat one first, treat the hypertension. Magnesium is not a panacea, but like potassium, magnesium should be a first-line therapy for most cases of hypertension. It is especially important for people taking diuretics, which wash out magnesium. Magnesium may also be helpful in reducing the risk of cardiac arrhythmias and sudden cardiac death. If you have mild-to-moderate hypertension, as 48 million Americans do, and you want to avoid medications, you may be able to do so with a heart-healthy diet, moderate weight loss (if needed), moderate exercise, adequate intake of potassium (which is plentiful in vegetables), moderate salt restriction, and supplementation with magnesium. Even if you do require medication, these steps will allow you to use lower doses and fewer drugs.

Because it is difficult to get enough magnesium even when you eat the right foods (beans, seafood, apricots, bananas, spinach, broccoli, sweet potatoes, seaweed, seeds), I recommend supplementation for most people. Start with 100 mg of magnesium twice daily with meals, then increase gradually. People who get diarrhea with standard magnesium oxide or other magnesium salts usually do fine with magnesium chelate. Absorption is best when magnesium is in solution (over-the-counter magnesium chloride solution), which makes it highly absorbable. Calcium-magnesium combinations are fine for healthy people, but for medical uses such as hypertension or migraines, magnesium may be more effective when taken alone than in multivitamins or in combination with other minerals.

Magnesium doses above the RDA should be taken with medical supervision. Seniors and people who have kidney disease or are taking medications for cardiovascular or neurological disorders should get medical supervision even for RDA doses.

As you can see, there is a lot more to maintaining cardiovascular health than taking statins. The body is an intricate, amazing balance of natural substances, and your health depends on providing your body with the essential nutrients it needs. Supplements are one way to provide vital nutrients. Foods are another, and selecting a heart-healthy diet for you is the subject of the next chapter.

10

Which Heart-Healthy Diet Is Right For You?
Your Individualized Optimum Diet

In a rational healthcare system, we would begin with nutrition, then natural therapies, and then drugs only when necessary. Today, it is usually just the opposite. Drugs have a role, absolutely, but they are frequently used first even when nutrition or natural remedies may be the answer.

—JAY S. COHEN, MD

A great number of people diagnosed medically with high cholesterol, "hypercholesterolemia," do not have medical disorders at all. They have nutritional imbalances. As a society, it is irrational for us to be elevating our LDL-C levels and triglyceride levels, while lowering HDL-C levels, with bad nutrition—then defining these abnormal measurements as medical disorders and taking powerful cholesterol-lowering drugs that have serious risks and cost billions, and all the while convincing ourselves that doing so is perfectly reasonable.

The preeminent role of good nutrition in reducing cardiovascular risk is not an alternative idea—it is emphasized in standard textbooks and drug references. Even package inserts and PDR descriptions of statin drugs acknowledge that diet comes first. For example, the dosage guidelines for Lipitor begin with: "The patient should be placed on a standard cholesterol-lowering diet before receiving Lipitor and should continue on this diet during treatment with Lipitor."[1] The American Hospital Formulary Service emphasizes the secondary role of statins to diet: "Statins are used as *adjuncts to dietary therapy* to reduce the risk of a first major acute coronary event."[2] (Emphasis added.)

Indeed, studies have shown that a good diet can reduce cholesterol levels as much as a moderate-dose statin drug.

More and more people are recognizing this and making changes in their diets, and manufacturers are responding with more healthful products (and a lot of junk products too). Overall, we have a long way to go. Just as with doctors' selections of prescription drugs, people's selections of foods are often more greatly influenced by intensive marketing than by medical science or common sense. Doctors say that many of their patients don't want to hear about changing their diets and would rather just pop a pill.

Although pills may reduce cholesterol levels, they do not correct the imbalances in people's systems that cause elevated cholesterol or CRP in the first place. Statins reduce cardiovascular risk 25 percent, which is good, but it is far from 100 percent. Thus, reducing cholesterol levels with statins is not the same as healing the system.

Even for people interested in healthier diets, it is less clear today than it was a decade ago what a healthy diet actually is. Ten years ago there was no doubt: a heart-healthy diet was a low-fat diet. Now this is not so certain. Low-carb diets have replaced low-fat ones as the new rage, different doctors advocate diametrically opposite approaches, different studies spew out conflicting results, and no one is quite sure what really works for whom. This ferment has its positive side and will undoubtedly lead to greater understanding and better methods, but for now it is creating a lot of confusion. Still, there are ways to identify the diet that is best for helping you maintain health and lower your risk of cardiovascular disease.

THE GREAT DEBATE: FATS VERSUS CARBOHYDRATES

The crux of the debate raging today centers on whether a low-fat or low-carbohydrate diet is best for reducing atherosclerosis and cardiovascular disease. In one corner we have Dr. Dean Ornish, the Pritikin Foundation, and the American Heart Association, which advocate low-fat diets. In the other corner we have Dr. Atkins advocates, Dr. Barry Sears, and many others who extol low-carbohydrate, high-fat diets. The debate is intense and important, yet to some degree it is absurd. The fact is, some fats are good and others are bad, and some carbohydrates are good and others are bad— and for most people, health depends more on choosing good fats and good carbohydrates than on strictly adhering to a rigid low-fat or low-carb doctrine. Moreover, no one diet works for everyone. As with drugs, individual variation is the critical factor with nutrition. Low-fat and low-carb diets can work, but the key question is: Which diet works for you? A doctor recently told me, "My friend went on the Atkins high-fat diet, and her cholesterol levels came way down. I went on the same diet, and my cholesterol levels went through the roof. Obviously, our systems work differently."

But the diet controversy makes good copy, sells millions of newspapers and magazines, and provides dynamic drama for television, so expect to hear plenty more from the Atkins and Ornish camps and anyone else with a study or opinion. It is interesting to hear these ideas, but always remember that as convincing as someone or some study may sound, it always comes down to your body type and tendencies.

It also ultimately comes down to calories. Whether you are on a low-fat or low-carb diet, if you eat too many calories, it will fail. You will gain weight, and your risk of heart attacks and strokes, as well as of diabetes and high blood pressure, will rise. "There is no magic combination of fat versus carbs versus protein," Dr. Alice Lichtenstein, a nutrition expert at Tufts University, told the Associated Press in 2002. "The bottom line is calories, calories, calories."[3] Actually, although I agree with her about calories, it does matter whether you choose a low-fat or low-carb diet. And there are ways of deciding which is best for you.

LOW-FAT DIETS

Atherosclerosis is infrequently hereditary in origin. Most of us get atherosclerosis because we consume too much fat, cholesterol, and calories.[4]

—DR. W.C. ROBERTS, *AMERICAN JOURNAL OF CARDIOLOGY*

In 1971, when I was a medical intern, I learned that my cholesterol was 265. I should not have been surprised, because my mother's family runs elevated cholesterol levels of 250 to 350 mg/dl, with too much of the bad LDL-C and too little of the good HDL-C. Since then, I have tried many diets. The Pritikin diet worked best, but it only reduced my cholesterol to 215—still too high. A doctor once recommended prescription drugs, but I declined. This was before statins, which I might have taken, but the drug he recommended was Lopid (gemfibrozil), and I was not impressed with its studies then. The studies showed that Lopid reduced cardiovascular death, but not overall death, so what was the point? Besides, although heart attacks and strokes killed most of my elderly relatives, they usually lived into their 70s or 80s, so I had time to try other things.

During the 1990s I developed a disabling vascular disorder and tried many things to get better. One of them was a vegetarian diet. I was not thinking about my cholesterol level then; I had more immediate problems. Eight months later, when I had some blood tests done, my cholesterol level was 165. I was shocked. I did not know that any diet could reduce cholesterol that much. For seven years now, with a modified vegetarian, low-fat diet, I have been able to keep my total cholesterol level in the 160 to 180 mg/dl range. People with family histories like mine are usually told that their cholesterol problems are genetic and that only prescription drugs will work. But "genetic" may not mean "impossible to do anything about." My genetic cholesterol disorder seemed intractable, but it actually meant that I simply could not handle bad fats. When I eat even small amounts of saturated or hydrogenated fats, my cholesterol and LDL-C levels skyrocket. Yet if I am a hawk about avoiding bad fats, my body does not become a cholesterol-manufacturing machine, and my cholesterol levels stay low.

This is not much different than the 40 percent reductions in LDL-C reported with the low-fat diet recommended by Dr. Dean Ornish, head of the Preventive Medicine Research Institute in Sausalito. "Most people can accomplish comparable reductions in LDL [to statins] by diet and lifestyle alone," stated Dr. Ornish.[5] One of the keys to the success of this approach is getting ample protein. When doing so, people report high levels of satiation and little problem with hunger.[6]

The extensive research on the heart-healthy Mediterranean diet demonstrates the same thing: *cholesterol problems are not due to the amount of fats people eat, but the types of fats.* Italians and Greeks eat as much fat as Americans, but their fat is primarily olive oil, which provides large amounts of heart-healthy monounsaturated fats. Olive oil also contains phenols that are similar to those found in green tea and red wine that inhibit LDL-C oxidation.[7] Thus, a study in *The New England Journal of Medicine* reported: "Greater adherence to the traditional Mediterranean diet is associated with a significant reduction in total mortality."[8]

The diet of the people of Okinawa, who have the longest life spans on the planet, contains high amounts of fat (from fish and soy) and carbohydrates (from vegetables and rice), but is low in saturated fats. Eskimos live on very high-fat foods, but Eskimos have low incidences of heart disease and arthritis because the fats they eat are very rich in omega-3 fatty acids.

The lesson is that Atkins, who stated "All fats are good," was wrong. Good fats are good, and bad fats are bad. Americans consume large quantities of bad fats—saturated fats and hydrogenated oils—that elevate cholesterol levels and cause cardiovascular disease. Indeed, every society that has adopted western dietary habits has suffered major increases in heart attacks and strokes. People from diet-healthy societies who come here and adopt our ways of eating get all of our diseases.

The trans fats—the "partially hydrogenated" oils so prevalent in processed foods—are a special problem. Dr. Walter Willett, one of America's foremost nutrition experts and a professor at the Harvard School of Public Health, states:

> Trans fats seem to be uniquely bad because they both raise LDL cholesterol, reduce HDL cholesterol, and also elevate lipoprotein A. There is no other type of fat that has that combination of adverse effects. Some people say that trans fats are only a small percentage of the diet, they are only on average 2–3% of the American diet. But there is no other artificial chemical in our food supply that comes anywhere near that level, and this level of intake could account for . . . 30,000 deaths a year. That is not a trivial number of premature deaths, and they are quite unnecessary.[9]

Margarine was created as a better alternative to saturated fat-laden butter. If margarines had been marketed in liquid form, allowing their oils to remain unsaturated, they might have been healthful. But in hardening the oils through hydrogenation so they would have the same consistency of butter, trans fatty acids were formed, and it has taken decades to learn that these are more destructive than the saturated fat they were designed to replace. Finally, to warn people about the dangers of trans fatty acids, the FDA now requires trans fats to be listed separately on food labels. The food industry resisted, of course, to their shame.

Advocates of low-fat diets with moderate amounts of protein and high-quality complex carbohydrates have plenty of evidence supporting their perspective. Studies repeatedly show that when people stick with low-fat diets, incidences of coronary disorders, heart attacks, and cardiac deaths plummet. Dr. Caldwell Esselstyn of the Cleveland Clinic reminds us that "although coronary artery disease is the leading killer of men and women in the USA, it is rarely encountered in cultures that base their nutrition primarily on grains, legumes, lentils, vegetables, and fruit."[10] In other words, the doctor is advocating a low-fat, moderate-protein—high-quality—diet based on natural foods. Dr. Dean Ornish has clearly demonstrated that for people with advanced coronary disease, strict restriction of fat, especially saturated and hydrogenated fat, can halt and sometimes reverse atherosclerosis.[11,12] A low-fat, high-quality diet does not mean going crazy on carbohydrates. It does not mean you can eat unlimited amounts of "low-fat" foods filled with sugars and calories. It does not mean breads and pastries made from refined white flour or loaded with sugar. Bad carbohydrates are just as bad as bad fats. You must select your carbohydrates just as carefully as you select fats.

· Most people do not have to adopt austere low-fat diets to obtain heart-healthy results. Good fats, particularly olive oil and adequate omega-3 oils, are healthful. For cooking, use olive oils or canola oil. Dr. Joe Mercola prefers coconut oil to canola, because coconut oil, although a saturated fat, has medicinal properties and does not break down with intense heat.

Good protein means fish, white-meat chicken and turkey, lean red meats, soy, beans, and egg whites. Protein and fat are additionally important because they are metabolized more slowly than carbohydrates, so they provide a sense of satiation that lasts many hours after meals. Meals with too few fats and proteins and too many carbohydrates, especially simple carbs like sugars and refined grains, can cause a return of hunger within a few hours after eating—and can raise insulin, triglyceride, and small particle LDL-C levels.

LOW-CARBOHYDRATE, HIGH-FAT DIETS

Advocates of low-carb, high-fat diets are correct in saying that when people, worried about eating too much fat, switch to low-fat and nonfat foods with more sugar and calories, they do themselves more harm than good. They are correct that too little fat in meals leads to less satiation and rebound hunger. But they are dead wrong when they go to the opposite extreme and claim that all carbohydrates, including complex carbohydrates filled with antioxidants and cancer-preventing substances, are bad and that saturated fat-laden meats, cream sauces, and lard are good. Yet the low-carb, high-fat fad is in full swing, and people are rushing to restaurants offering fat-laden fare. This trend will take us back to the 1950s, when similar diets triggered an epidemic of heart attacks and strokes.

Some people can handle low-carb, high-fat diets, but not high-carb diets. A high intake of poor-quality carbohydrates leads to elevated levels of glucose, insulin, and triglycerides, and reduced levels of HDL-C—a destructive combination known as *syndrome X* (or the *metabolic syndrome*). The tendency toward syndrome X is genetically determined. Syndrome X has been recognized by integrative physicians for years and is finally being recognized by mainstream medicine.

This recognition has followed several decades during which concerns about fats led manufacturers to produce and people to eat foods filled with simple, nutrient-deficient carbohydrates—sugars and white flour—with more calories than the foods they replaced. The result is that since the 1980s, we have seen burgeoning increases in obesity and obesity-related illnesses such as diabetes and high blood pressure. From the 1970s to 1999, obesity increased from 15 percent to 27 percent in the U.S. Today, more than 30 percent of Americans are obese and nearly two-thirds are overweight. The most common culprit: bad carbohydrates—but not all carbohydrates.

Syndrome X is characterized by reduced insulin sensitivity, which is also known as insulin resistance: the inability of a person's cells to respond properly to the insulin that is secreted by the pancreas in response to the carbohydrates eaten. People with normal insulin sensitivity can metabolize carbohydrates properly. When insulin sensitivity is reduced, cells are less able to utilize glucose, and blood glucose levels rise. To compensate, more insulin is produced, but the tissues can become even more insulin resistant, and more and more carbohydrate is converted into fat. People become overweight or obese, which worsens the process. By eating properly and not becoming overweight, many people with a genetic tendency toward syndrome X can avoid the development of the syndrome.

Prevention is key because the progression of syndrome X leads to its typical features: abdominal obesity, elevated triglycerides, low HDL-C, elevated blood pressure, and an elevated fasting blood glucose level. This is serious—syndrome X is associated with a five- to nine-fold increased risk of diabetes and a two- to three-fold increased risk of cardiovascular mortality.[13] This is why Dr. Jonathan Wright recommends: "If you have type 2 diabetes or symptoms of low blood sugar, or if these problems are in your family, then a low-carb diet probably is your best choice."[14]

About 23 percent of the population has syndrome X.[15] In a recent survey of sixty year-olds, 42 percent had diagnosable metabolic syndromes.[16] Integrative practitioners report even higher percentages in their practices. "About 60 percent of the patients I see have syndrome X," Dr. Ron Hoffman, former president of the American College for the Advancement of Medicine, told me. "Of course, my population may be skewed by the kinds of people who decide to see me."[17]

"I see a lot of syndrome X patients," says Dr. Jeffrey Baker, MD. "Insulin plays a big role in the elevated cholesterol of many of my patients. Controlling excess carbohydrates is key. The diet I recommend includes clean, lean protein including some meats, avoidance of simple sugars and simple carbohydrates, and moderate exercise."[18]

Dr. Baker makes the key distinction between simple and complex carbohydrates. Simple carbohydrates are quickly converted to glucose and cause quick spikes in insulin levels. Simple carbohydrates include not only sugar and honey, but also potatoes, white rice, and the refined wheat or corn flour found in most breads, crackers, pasta, tortillas, and snacks. Flour, even enriched flour, is quickly broken down into simple sugars and acts just like them. People with syndrome X can eat fruits, but only in moderation because of their high content of fructose, a simple sugar. But fruit is far better than a candy bar or a muffin. Fruit juices are taboo, just as any sweetened beverages are for syndrome Xers. Low-carb foods that are high in alcohols allow manufacturers to claim "low net carbohydrates," but are also discouraged because alcohols are handled similiar to carbohydrates by the body.

Results with low-carb diets can sometimes be dramatic. An integrative doctor told me of an overweight, middle-aged man with a cholesterol level above 250, and triglyceride and blood glucose levels sky high—above 400 and 300, respectively—a classic syndrome X. In fact, these numbers were an improvement: they were worse before the man's mainstream doctor placed him on a statin, and Lopid (to lower triglycerides), and a diabetes drug. The integrative doctor, who is also a board-certified internist, analyzed the man's diet, which contained a lot of refined grains and tons of pasta. By limiting the refined grains and modestly increasing the protein and good oils, the man's blood studies returned to normal within months and he was able to discontinue the drugs.

This is an extreme case, of course, and unless you have diabetes or syndrome X, or tendencies toward these, you do not have to adopt an austere low-carb diet to maintain health. This is why I cringed when I heard Dr. Atkins say flatly, "Fats are good, carbohydrates are bad." Lard is not healthy. Highly saturated fats are not healthy. There may be some people who can handle bad fats, but not the majority, and certainly not in their everyday diets. And although some people using the Atkins diet do not get elevations in their cholesterol levels, this does not mean that this diet is healthy in the long run.

The effects of the Atkins diet were underscored in two studies.[19,20] In the studies, people on the Atkins diet for six months lost more weight than those on a low-fat diet. This may be because the high-fat diet worked better, but it may also be because there is a greater initial loss of water from people's tissues with the Atkins diet—a loss that returns later, because at twelve months, the difference in the two diets was insignificant. The media, as expected, trumpeted the better short-term weight loss with the Atkins diet and the better HDL-C and triglyceride numbers in Atkins dieters. But it conveniently overlooked the fact that LDL-C levels did not drop in the Atkins group, yet did drop in the low-fat group. And there were other concerns with the Atkins diet, as one of the studies described:

> The low-carbohydrate diet [Atkins diet] was associated with a greater improvement in some risk factors for coronary heart disease (serum triglycerides and serum HDL cholesterol), but not others (blood pressure, insulin sensitivity, and serum LDL cholesterol). It is also possible that the large amount of saturated fats and small amounts of fruits, vegetables, and fiber consumed during the low-carbohydrate diet can independently increase the risk of coronary heart disease.[18]

I do credit Dr. Atkins for sticking to his guns under intense criticism in order to make two important points. First, *some* people do not do well on low-fat diets. Carbohydrate addiction is a reality for some people. Meals should include some high-quality fats and protein. Second, *some* fat is necessary for a lasting sense of satiation after meals, thereby turning off the hunger signal and allowing people to snack less and reduce overall calories. In this vein, the recent studies on the Atkins diet showed that it worked not because it altered people's metabolism, as Atkins thought, but because people simply ate fewer calories.

It is also important to note that in the long-term maintenance phase of the Atkins diet, vegetables are encouraged. Indeed, the Atkins people recently adjusted their guidelines to include more vegetables. That is because vegetables, with their complex carbohydrates and antioxidants, remain a cornerstone of any healthy diet and can fill you up with relatively few calories. And the fact is, the single most important thing syndrome Xers can do is maintain a healthy weight. The single most important thing that overweight syndrome Xers can do is lose weight.

One of the best ways to lose weight is to get more bang for your calories. *The Wall Street Journal* article "The Diet That Works" listed many practical strategies for losing weight. One of the best was to "eat big food," foods that provide a lot of volume for their calories.[21] People tend to eat the same volume of food each day, and soups, vegetables, and fruits provide the greatest volume for the least calories. In contrast, the article noted that a single soda contains 150 calories, which is a lot of calories for the volume. If you normally drink one soda a day, replacing the soda with bottled water every day for a year can produce a loss of 15 pounds. (For every ten calories you cut every day for a year, you will lose one pound.)

The current fad toward fats and against carbohydrates has given vegetables like carrots a bad rap, because they measure poorly on a scale known as the *glycemic index*. This index was developed to measure the impact of a food on insulin levels. Unfortunately, the methodology of the glycemic index is flawed, and newer studies using the *glycemic load* scale reveal that carrots, as well as whole fruits (apples, pears, peaches, berries, etc.), are indeed healthful.[22] Yet, some experts still use the outdated glycemic index and arrive at questionable results. "If you look at tables of glycemic index, you will see things that should bother an intelligent person," states Dr. Gabe Mirkin. "A carrot has almost the same glycemic index as sugar does. This is ridiculous. A carrot is far safer for diabetics than table sugar."[23] Tables listing the glycemic load of common foods can be found at the websites of *Consumer Reports* and the Harvard Medical School. A very complete list was published in the *American Journal of Clinical Nutrition* in 2002 (volume 76, pages 5–56).

Moreover, foods must be considered in the context of the other foods with which they are eaten. Pasta is a high glycemic-load food, but this is partially mitigated when pasta is eaten with olive oil-rich sauces and a salad full of complex carbohydrates. The greater problem by far is the plethora of sodas, candies, sugars, and refined-flour breads, pastries, pancakes, doughnuts, and crackers that are eaten alone or with other refined carbohydrate products. The morning doughnut-and-coffee-with-sugar routine is a typical, harmful refined-carbohydrate fix that drives insulin levels up and contributes to the syndrome X phenomenon.

GRAINS: THE WHOLE STORY

Recent epidemiological data indicate that diets rich in high-fiber whole grains are associated with lower risk of coronary heart disease (CHD) and type 2 [adult onset] diabetes mellitus. These data are consistent with results from recent metabolic experiments suggesting favorable lipid profiles and glycemic control associated with higher intake of whole grains, but not with refined grains. It seems prudent, therefore, to distinguish whole-grain rather than refined-grain cereal products for the prevention of chronic diseases.[24]

—JOURNAL OF THE AMERICAN COLLEGE OF NUTRITION

Some low-carb, high-fat advocates warn people against eating any types of grains, which are a carbohydrate-rich food. Their warnings might be appropriate for people with diabetes, but not for most people. The problem with breads and pasta today is not that they are grains, but that 95 percent of them are refined instead of whole grains. Other anti-grain advocates claim that people do best on the foods on which the human species evolved through the eons, and they tout the Neanderthal diet. This does not include grains, which only became part of the human diet around 3,000 B.C., so grains just cannot be good. But just because something is new does not mean it is bad. Sanitation, electricity, and temperature-controlled homes were not part of our natural heritage either, but I tend to believe they are changes for the better. So are whole grains.

Some warn that grains are bad because many people cannot handle the gluten contained in wheat. This is true for some people, and an elimination diet to identify food intolerances to gluten-containing grains such as wheat (including durum, semolina, spelt, kamut), rye, barley, and oats has merit for people with chronic disorders. However, rice and corn do not contain gluten and needn't be avoided, nor do buckwheat, millet, amaranth, soy, or teff flours.

Other grain foes argue that grains have a high glycemic index and are quickly digested into glucose, pushing blood glucose levels and insulin production way up, producing syndrome X. But not everyone is prone to syndrome X, and although refined grains may catapult insulin levels, whole grains don't. An article in the *American Journal of Clinical Nutrition* explained:

> During the past decade, several lines of evidence have collectively provided strong support for a relation between diets and diabetes incidence. In diabetic patients, evidence from medium-term studies suggests that replacing high-glycemic-index carbohydrates with low-glycemic-index foods will improve glycemic control and, among persons treated with insulin, will reduce hypoglycemic episodes. These dietary changes, which can be made by replacing products made with white flour and potatoes with whole-grain, minimally refined cereal products, have also been associated with a lower risk of cardiovascular disease and can be an appropriate component of recommendations for an overall healthy diet.[25]

As demonstrated in the inset on page 142, study after study has proven that whole grains are associated with less cardiovascular disease and diabetes. Refined grains are quickly digested and impact the body like sugars, but whole grains with their complex structures and high concentrations of fiber, protein, and antioxidants are digested much more slowly. Refined grains cause insulin levels to spike; whole grains don't.

Whole Grains, Diabetes, and Cancer

Here is a small sample of the many articles in the medical literature about the benefits of whole-grain foods.

■ *American Journal of Clinical Nutrition:* "Whole grains can provide a substantial contribution to the improvement of the diets of Americans. A number of whole grain foods and grain fiber sources are beneficial in reduction of insulin resistance and improvement in glucose tolerance. Dietary recommendations of health organizations suggest consumption of three servings a day of whole grain foods; however, Americans generally fall below this standard."[26]

■ *American Journal of Clinical Nutrition:* "Consistent findings from prospective studies of diverse populations and supporting data from metabolic trials strongly support the premise that an increased intake of whole-grain foods can lower the risk of type 2 diabetes."[27]

■ *American Journal of Public Health:* "These findings suggest that substituting whole- for refined-grain products may decrease the risk of diabetes mellitus."[28]

■ *Journal of the American College of Nutrition:* "Dietary guidance recommends consumption of whole grains for the prevention of cancer. Epidemiologic studies find that whole grains are protective against cancer, especially gastrointestinal cancers such as gastric and colonic, and hormonally-dependent cancers including breast and prostate."[29]

■ *Nutrition and Metabolism in Cardiovascular Disease:* "Whole grain food intake was consistently related to reduced risk of several types of cancer, particularly of the upper digestive tract neoplasms. Epidemiological evidence of the relation between fiber and colorectal cancer indicate possible protections. In contrast, refined grain intake was associated to increased risk of different types of cancer, pointing to a potential role of insulin-like growth factor 1."[30]

One of the latest studies, from Boston's Brigham and Women's Hospital and the Harvard Medical School, was published in the *American Journal of Clinical Nutrition*. This was a prospective study, which is one of the most powerful types of clinical studies, following 86,190 male doctors for five years. Comparing matched groups that differed only in their intake of refined versus whole grains, the study found:

Both total mortality and cardiovascular disease mortality-specific mortality were inversely associated with whole-grain but not refined-grain breakfast cereal intake. These prospective data highlight the importance of distinguishing whole-grain from refined-grain cereals in the prevention of chronic diseases.[31]

Indeed, in an earlier study in the same journal, people who ate cereals, muffins, spaghetti, breads and rolls—and even chocolate chip cookies—made with whole grains had reduced after-meal and fasting insulin levels. Of course, when made with refined grains, these foods cause insulin levels to spike. But in this study, even in overweight subjects, who usually have even greater insulin spiking, the whole-grain foods produced improved insulin response. This study, backed by extensive epidemiologic evidence, showed that there is an "inverse association between consumption of cereal fiber or whole grains and type 2 diabetes, cardiovascular disease, and total mortality."[32]

Just as olive and omega-3 oils have far different effects on human physiology and health than saturated and hydrogenated fats, whole grains have far different effects than refined grains and other simple carbohydrates. Epidemiologic studies involving tens of thousands of people have repeatedly shown reduced risks of heart attacks in people consuming whole grains. Other studies have shown that whole grains reduce cancer risks.

"Whole grains are rich sources of a wide range of phytochemicals with anticarcinogenic properties," Dr. Joanne Slavin, Professor of Food and Nutrition at the University of Minnesota, told *The New York Times.* "Some of these phytochemicals block DNA damage and suppress cancer cell growth."[33] They are also a rich source of minerals that are deficient in many diets. For example, a half-cup of white rice contains only 4 mg of magnesium, but the same amount of brown rice contains 47 mg. A slice of white bread contains 6 mg of magnesium, yet whole-wheat bread contains 24 mg.[34]

The benefits of whole grains are so well proven, the FDA allows food manufacturers to trumpet their benefits on their packaging:

> Diets rich in whole-grain foods and other plant foods low in total fat, saturated fat and cholesterol, may help reduce the risk of heart disease and certain cancers.[33]

The evidence is overwhelming: whole grains are beneficial for most people. Some diets such as Dr. Mercola's *No-Grain Diet* recommend avoidance of all grains during the early phases of treatment of carbohydrate addiction. A small percentage of people may be so sensitive to any carbohydrates that grains of any kind are a problem. But for most people, whole grains have a well-deserved place as one of the cornerstones of a healthy diet.

The recommended daily amount of grains is six to eleven servings, so grains are an important food group. Whole-grain breads, cereals, and even pasta are so plentiful today, it is easy to find tasty products. But be sure to check the ingredients, because many products boasting "whole grains" are not entirely whole-grained, but in fact contain mostly white flour. Fortunately, food manufacturers are gradually conforming to consumers' demand for fully whole-grain products. It is time for you to replace the refined grains in your diet with whole grains.

WHICH DIET IS BEST FOR YOU?

It is unfortunate that while western science has greatly increased our understanding of human physiology and nutrition in recent decades, our everyday nutrition has become increasingly filled with harmful and unnatural foods that have caused epidemics of obesity, hypercholesterolemia, hypertension and other cardiovascular disease, syndrome X, and diabetes. The origins of this paradox are not hard to discover. During the twentieth century, major changes were made in food production without any consideration for their long-term effects. Western diets veered from natural foods to manufactured products based on shelf life, taste, and salesmanship. Whole grains were replaced with refined grains. Healthy oils were replaced with hydrogenated oils. Sugar use skyrocketed. It was a recipe for disaster.

Our sources of animal protein saw dramatic changes, too. In previous centuries, humans ate animals that grazed on grasses instead of being fattened on grains. When raised on grasses, animals develop high levels of heart-healthy omega-3 oils and less saturated fat. In the twentieth century, we got the saturated fat (and hormones and antibiotics) with little omega-3 oil from our animal products.

Food manufacturers also learned that products filled with fats and sugars taste and smell better and are nearly irresistible. Intensive advertising on television and in the print media lulled us into believing food selection is all about taste, not health. The food industry created and catered to this new taste-fixated market. The results of all of these changes have been obvious since the 1950s, and we have been trying to find our way out ever since. First, low-fat, high-carb diets became the way. Now the pendulum is swinging to the other extreme of low-carb, high-fat diets. Just the other day I saw an advertisement from a fast food company proclaiming its new low-carb breakfast: hamburger, cheese, bacon, and refined flour bun. "Only 5 grams of carbs" it boasted while not mentioning the frightening amount of saturated fat. Such foods will take us right back to the high-fat heart disease epidemics of the mid twentieth century.

So which is the villain: fats or carbohydrates? My answer is simple:

- *Bad fats (saturated and hydrogenated fats) are bad.*

- *Good fats (olive oil, omega-3 fatty acids, canola oil for cooking) are good.*

- *Bad carbohydrates (simple sugars, processed flour) are bad.*

- *Good carbohydrates (complex carbohydrates as in vegetables, fruit, and whole grains) are good.*

You do not have to become carbo-phobic or fat-phobic to eat right. Human bodies need fat, carbohydrate, and protein. What is the right balance? Which diet—low-fat or low-carb—is best for you? For most people, the answer lies between the two extremes of Atkins and Ornish: a balanced diet based on healthful foods. Neither an extreme low-fat nor extreme low-carb diet is necessary or desirable for cardiovascular health in most cases. The best diets contain good fats, good carbohydrates, and good protein—lean, clean protein, as Dr. Baker puts it in a healthful balance. The best diets are based on olive oil, omega-3 oils, vegetables, whole grains, fruit, nuts, legumes, fish, chicken, lean meats, and low-fat or non-fat dairy. These are the pillars of the Mediterranean diet, the DASH diet that has been proven to reduce high blood pressure, and to a large extent the Okinawan diet and, more recently, the Zone diets and the South Beach diet.

Indeed, both the Ornish and Atkins approaches recommend many of these same foods. This really is not surprising, because the foundations of a heart-healthy diet are clear, as described by nationally recognized experts Drs. Frank Hu and Walter Willett:

> Substantial evidence indicates that diets using non-hydrogenated unsaturated fats as the predominant form of dietary fat, whole grains as the main form of carbohydrates, an abundance of fruits and vegetables, and adequate omega-3 fatty acids can offer significant protection against coronary heart disease. Such diets, together with regular physical activity, avoidance of smoking, and maintenance of a healthy body weight, may prevent the majority of cardiovascular disease in western populations.[35]

It can be helpful to know whether your metabolism runs better with a higher ratio of fats or carbohydrates. A new method for doing so is *metabolic typing*. This approach, based on the book *The Metabolic Typing Diet* by Wolcott and Fahey,[36] measures many different factors in determining your physiological and psychological tendencies and the diet that fits your profile the best. Wolcott's work is based on studies and writings that go back a century. The book offers a test that defines your best diet. Although I think the test requires refinement, the basic tenets of the book are sound, and I agree with Wolcott's main theme: different people do well on different food balances. Or, in Wolcott's words:

> Standardized nutritional approaches fail to recognize that, for genetic reasons, people are all very different from one another on a biochemical or metabolic level. Due to widely varying hereditary influences, we all process or utilize foods and nutrients very differently. Thus, the very same nutritional protocol that enables one person to lead a long healthy life full of robust health can cause serious illness in someone else. As the ancient Roman philosopher Lucretius once said, 'One man's food is another's poison.' It turns out his statement is quite literally true.[37]

If you have elevated cholesterol, CRP, or other risk factors, you may have to work with a health professional. Because diet is so key to treating these conditions, you should seek a practitioner who understands not only the importance of diet, but also that different people do well with different approaches. Start with a low-fat, low-carb, or a balanced carb-fat-protein diet and monitor its effect on your cholesterol, triglyceride, LDL-C particle size, and glucose levels. If the first diet does not produce the desired results, try another. In this way, it is easy to identify the diet that is best for you. What you eat is either facilitating health or fueling disease. Most people with elevated cholesterol or syndrome X have eaten their way to their disorders. Although I did not know it, I certainly ate my way to my cholesterol problem, and now I have eaten my way out of it. Now I load each meal with several low-calorie, high-volume vegetables, with good oils, protein, whole grains, and a piece of fruit—a diet that allows me to maintain a low cholesterol and proper weight while never feeling hungry.

People repeatedly tell me that they hate taking medication. Most people with high cholesterol, high triglycerides, elevated homocysteine, or syndrome X do not have to take medication. You do not have to become one of the 62 percent of the population who is overweight, or one of the 50 percent of Americans who develop advanced atherosclerosis and coronary symptoms,[4] or one of the 90 percent who ultimately develop high blood pressure. You and your children do not have to be among the burgeoning numbers of diabetics.

Identify your metabolic type, adopt the proper diet, orient your meals to high-volume, low-calorie foods, and monitor the results. If a low-fat diet causes problems, add more healthy fats and reduce the carbs, especially the simple carbs. If a low-carb diet causes your cholesterol levels to jump, switch to a low-fat, high complex-carbohydrate approach. Balance these diets with enough protein. Keep your weight down. Some experts believe that it does not really matter which diet you use as long as it helps you maintain a healthy weight. Find the diet that works best for you and stick to it. Commit yourself to it. You only get one body. Treat it like it's important to you.

A LITTLE EXERCISE MAKES A BIG DIFFERENCE

You already know that exercise is important. You know that our bodies are biologically designed for activity, and that our current culture of inactivity is unnatural. Indeed, exercise is so important that it is better to be somewhat overweight and exercising than to be at a good weight and not exercising.

"Of all the behaviors that are health related, physical activity is by far the most important," Dr. Tim Byers, professor of preventive medicine at the University of Colorado School of Medicine in Denver and co-chairman of the American Cancer Society's cancer prevention guideline committee, told *USA Today*. "It's strongly protective for heart disease, diabetes and some types of cancer, and regular physical activity is essential for a lifetime of weight control."[38] This is not a minority position. "The best alternative method is exercise, which reduces cardiac mortality 50% (much better than statins) and reduces overall mortality as well," stated Dr. Wayne Anderson, Chairman of Family Practice and the Preventive Health Task Force, Scripps Clinic, at a recent conference.

You do not have to overdo it to obtain benefits from exercise. Studies show that just a little exercise a day is nearly as effective for maintaining health as triathlon training. Thirty to forty-five minutes a day is enough. Yet fewer than 50 percent of Americans get thirty minutes of exercise a day. The most common excuse is, "I can't find the time to exercise." No doubt, with so many people working fifty to sixty hours a week these days, it is difficult. Here is a suggestion if you cannot find the time to exercise: get a treadmill or exercise bike, place it in your den and use it in the evening when you watch television or read. By combining exercise with other routine activities, it does not take any extra time from other obligations, and exercise passes quickly while watching TV or a movie. If you are older or have medical problems, check with your doctor before starting an exercise regimen.

Start gradually in order to avoid quick burnout. Don't push it. It is better to exercise at a low, comfortable intensity for thirty to sixty minutes than at high intensity for short, unpleasant durations. You will enjoy it more, and with consistency your strength and endurance will increase naturally and make more strenuous workouts easy. Surprisingly quickly, exercise will make you feel stronger, healthier, fit, better in every way.

11

How To Cut Statin Costs by Fifty Percent or More

Precision prescribing is not much help if you cannot afford the medication in the first place. Sometimes treatment decisions must be made not only on what is best, but also on what is affordable. More than 40 percent of Americans lack health insurance. Millions more lack adequate drug coverage. Cost, unfortunately, is often the deciding issue not only of which medication will be used, but whether any treatment can be used at all. Even people with traditionally good prescription drug coverage are finding it increasingly difficult to pay for their prescriptions as insurers charge higher and higher copayments. Copayments of $75 are not unusual for brand-name drugs. Some people must pay $500 or more each year for pharmaceuticals before their insurance pays a dime.

This is occurring because insurers are beset by ever-escalating drug costs. Although large insurance companies and HMOs can make special arrangements with drug companies by buying in quantity, drug costs continue to be the fastest rising cost for insurers and healthcare systems. Drug companies reap 15 percent to 20 percent profit increases and lead the Fortune 500 year after year, even during recessions that reduce other industries' profits to nil. Someone is paying for these profits. That someone is you and me and our health systems and insurers. Indeed, prescription drug prices have escalated so much, they cost some health organizations more than all of their patients' visits to doctors or all of their patients' hospitalizations combined.

WHY PRESCRIPTION DRUG PRICES ARE SO HIGH

Why do drugs cost so much? How can the drug industry resist market econ-

omies and buck economic downturns? How can drug companies keep
increasing the prices of drugs when the research that produced these same
drugs was paid for years ago?

A Monopolistic Market

The medication market is not an open market. It is a monopolistic market. When the
government grants a patent for a new drug, it gives the manufacturer a
monopoly that lasts seventeen years. The patents in themselves are not the
entire problem. Drug companies require patents to ensure adequate returns on
their investments. Yet the patents also provide the basis for which a combination of economic factors allows drug companies to charge whatever they want.

Consumers Have No Power

You may be paying the bill and taking the risk, but you do not decide which
drug and dosage you will get. Unlike buying cars or clothing or other com-
modities where you make the final decisions, you are a passive recipient in
the medication marketplace. This is because doctors, not patients, decide
which drugs patients take. Doctors are the gatekeepers. Because doctors
determine which drugs will be blockbusters and which will be busts, drug
companies target most of their marketing to doctors. That is why stronger
doses and simple dosing regimens are the rule, because that is what many
doctors prefer. If you ask doctors about this, they usually deny it, but their
prescribing patterns are clear. In fact, they are closely monitored by the drug
industry, which buys access to pharmacy records of doctors' prescribing
patterns. Drug companies know what doctors choose, and they eagerly
provide what doctors prefer.

Doctors Are Inadequately Informed About Drug Costs

Traditionally, doctors paid little attention to drug costs. Today, many doctors are more cognizant of this issue, but it is difficult for doctors to keep
track of the prices of each and every drug that they prescribe. Moreover,
drug prices differ greatly from one pharmacy to another, and different
patients have different drug coverages. Doctors have enough trouble trying
to diagnose, treat, and answer the questions of their patients in the limited
time allowed. Cost is left up to you. If you have cost constraints or limited
coverage, you have to speak up. That is what Tables 11.1 and 11.2 are for—
to allow you and your doctor to compare statin costs quickly and make
decisions accordingly.

Doctors have another consideration: Choosing the drug they think will work best for you. This is the doctor's first concern, as it should be. Drug companies know this and apply all of their means—advertising, drug reps, free seminars, and drug samples, amounting to $15,000 per doctor per year—to convince doctors that their statin is better than their competitors' statins. The companies emphasize effectiveness, not cost. Drug companies know that if a doctor is convinced that one statin is truly superior, that is what he or she will likely choose regardless of the cost.

Consumers Cannot Bargain Shop

With other products, you can shop around until you find the best buy. You can, for example, compare the costs of a Ford, Toyota, Chrysler, and Chevy and take your pick. But once your doctor writes a prescription for Zocor, you cannot tell the pharmacist to give you Mevacor or Pravachol instead. Prescriptions are orders, and you have to follow them.

Medication Purchases Are Not Elective

Drug manufacturers know that patients are a captive audience. You can decide to buy a new car or stereo or dress now or next month or next year, but if you are in pain or have a disorder that must be treated, you need that prescription now. Most people do not take medication because they want to, but because they have to. So you cannot walk away, no matter the cost. You will get the drug your doctor prescribes at the cost the manufacturer demands, whether you like it or not. In other words, your concerns can be ignored. That is why drug companies can get away with charging such high prices, just as they get away with ignoring lower, safer doses that millions of people would like to have.

HOW TO OBTAIN SUBSTANTIAL SAVINGS WITH STATINS

People and healthcare systems can do a lot to reduce the cost of treating elevated cholesterol or C-reactive protein. Here are some possibilities.

Discuss The Costs With Your Doctor

Most patients do not ask about costs when their doctors write prescriptions. People rarely ask doctors about the comparative costs of statins or any drugs. They should. If enough people start asking, doctors will start to inquire. This is the first step toward reversing the current system and toward making manufacturers aware that doctors do care about price and will make some choices based on it. Make a copy of the tables in this chapter for yourself and for your doctor, so he or she can consider costs with you and with others as well.

Compare Pharmacy Prices

Prices between chain pharmacies can vary a bit, sometimes enough to make a special trip worthwhile. Discount stores can sometimes save you a lot more. Also check internet pharmacies and websites of Canadian pharmacies providing drugs at government-controlled prices. Table 11.1 compares the prices at a local chain pharmacy and Costco for a commonly prescribed dosage of each statin. As you can see, there is quite a difference.

TABLE 11.1 COMPARATIVE COSTS OF STATIN DRUGS		
Prices for 100 pills of various statin medications at a chain pharmacy and at Costco in Southern California, August 2003.		
STATIN DRUG	PHARMACY CHAIN	COSTCO
Lovastatin (generic Mevacor) 20 mg	$265	$ 63
Lescol 40 mg	$214	$162
Lipitor 10 mg	$262	$206
Mevacor 20 mg	$292	$223
Pravachol 40 mg	$422	$374
Zocor 20 mg	$425	$385

Consider Generics

Now that lovastatin, the generic of Mevacor, is available, it should make a big difference. "Mevacor is plenty powerful for most patients," David Campen, Kaiser's medical director of drug-use management, told the *Wall Street Journal*. "It will work for the vast majority of people with high cholesterol, at a cost that is far more affordable."[1] But will it make a difference? In mid-2003, the price of 100 tablets of generic 20-mg lovastatin at my local chain pharmacy was a disappointing $265, only about 10 percent less than Mevacor itself at $292 and still higher than some equivalent statins. Yet at Costco, 100 tablets of 20-mg lovastatin was $63, a huge savings.

If your health insurance includes prescription drug coverage, you can save a lot even at your local pharmacy. Many insurers charge very low copayments for generic drugs. Your copayment for generic lovastatin may be $15 instead of $75 for a brand-name statin.

Over-the-counter statins may soon offer another low-dose, lower-cost alternative. In Britain, Zocor can now be bought without a prescription. The dosage is 10 mg. Over-the-counter statins may offer a price advantage for people who pay for statins out of their own pockets, but it may lead health-care insurers to refuse to cover subscribers who require only modest statin doses. In addition, there are legitimate concerns that people using over-the-counter statins will not get adequate supervision to ensure the medication is having the desired effect on cholesterol or CRP, and that the drug is not causing liver inflammation or other metabolic problems.

Consider The Every-Other-Day Approach

If your doctor wants you to take 20 mg of Lipitor every day, ask about taking 40 mg every other day (see Chapter 4 for a discussion of this approach). The effects on cholesterol and C-reactive protein levels should be about the same. If the 40-mg dose is not too strong for you, the cost difference is considerable: 100 tablets of 20-mg Lipitor cost $301, whereas 50 tablets of 40-mg Lipitor cost $152. Spread over a year, that is a $600 savings.

Consider Other Alternatives

Many doctors consider niacin as effective as statins in reducing cholesterol and LDL-C. Moreover, niacin is more effective than statins in raising HDL-C, a primary risk factor for women as well as for men with low HDL-C levels. Niacin also reduces elevated levels of lipoprotein A and small particle LDL, although it may not lower CRP as well as statins do. Some doctors choose niacin before statins for many of their patients. Some brands of intermediate-acting niacin are much less expensive than brand-name statins. Inositol hexanicotinate, which many alternative doctors prefer, is available on the shelf and is very inexpensive.

LOWER DOSES COST LESS

Lower statin doses are not only safer, but cheaper (see Table 11.2). At Costco, 100 tablets of Lipitor 40 mg cost $303; 10 mg costs $206. One hundred tablets of Zocor 40 mg cost $386; 10 mg costs $226; 5 mg costs $171.

What if you require greater LDL-C reductions than these lower doses provide? Statins should not be the only thing you do to reduce cholesterol or CRP. A heart-healthy diet is always the most important strategy of all and can have as much impact as a moderate-dose statin. And you can use supplements such as plant sterols that block cholesterol absorption. These products are much cheaper, and work as well as similar-acting prescription drugs, Welchol or Zetia, which doctors frequently prescribe with statins. You can also try soy and garlic, which have modest abilities to reduce cholesterol.

Another way to reduce costs is by buying larger pills and splitting them. This is most easily done with Lipitor, Mevacor, and Pravachol. Some doctors and pharmacists encourage pill splitting, but others do not, so I always advise getting your own doctor's opinion. Usually it does not matter whether the pills split exactly evenly. Because statins are long-acting drugs, their effects remain fairly constant even if you take a little more on one day and a little less on the next.

If you are taking capsules, splitting the pill is not an option. However, for a fee, some compounding pharmacies can make lower-dose versions of capsule medications if your doctor writes an order. If you or your doctor do not have a local compounding pharmacy, the Professional Compounding Centers of America (800-331-2498; 281-933-6948) will help you find one.

SAVING MONEY BY USING NATURAL PRODUCTS WITH OR INSTEAD OF STATINS

In general, natural products are much cheaper than prescription statins (see Table 11.3). Of course, prices can vary greatly between brands, and the quality of supplements is a concern. Studies have repeatedly shown that many supplements, albeit less than the majority, do not contain the amounts claimed on their labels. The FDA is now cracking down on supplement manufacturers, and hopefully this will provide greater standardization and reliability. However, this improved reliability may have a cost. High-quality, pharmaceutical-grade supplements can be more expensive.

For example, one internet supplement manufacturer offers ninety tablets of policosanol for $16. In contrast, sixty 10-mg tablets of standardized, pharmaceutical-grade policosanol from the Life Extension Foundation cost $47 ($35 for members). The price drops to about $31 if you buy six bottles ($24 for members).

The best known brand-name form of red yeast rice is Cholestin, for which one internet supplier charges $63 for 120 capsules, containing 600 mg each. The price drops to about $45 each if you buy six bottles for $278. These prices are much higher than generic products from lesser known companies, which charge less than $20, but even the prices of Cholestin are substantially lower than brand-name statins.

TABLE 11.2   COMPARATIVE COSTS OF VARIOUS STATIN DOSES

This cost comparison is based on prices listed at the Costco pharmacy website, January 2005.

Generic Lovastatin	Mevacor
10 mg: $36	10 mg: $129
20 mg: $56	20 mg: $221
40 mg: $98	40 mg: $402

Crestor	Pravachol
5 mg: $245	10 mg: $294
10 mg: $248	20 mg: $292
20 mg: $248	40 mg: $419
40 mg: $249	80 mg: $427

Lescol	Zocor
20 mg: $186	5 mg: $181
40 mg: $188	10 mg: $243
80 mg: $232	20 mg: $412

Lipitor	
10 mg: $232	40 mg: $412
20 mg: $322	80 mg: $431
40 mg: $323	
80 mg: $327	

A price comparison of prescription Niaspan and its alternative medicine counterpart, inositol nicotinate, is an eye-opener that should motivate healthcare systems and insurers to take a closer look at this nonprescription alternative. Prescription Niaspan, 1,000 mg, costs $206 for 100 tablets; inositol nicotinate, 500 mg, costs $20.

MAKING THE DECISION

Ultimately, treatment decisions should always be based on what will work best for you. For most people there is not much difference between the benefits of one statin versus another, so it is reasonable to consider cost factors. If enough doctors and patients do this, perhaps the pharmaceutical industry will finally have to heed market influences. That would be a boon for individuals and families (drug costs, insurance premiums), doctors, pharmacies, hospitals, nursing homes, insurers, governments—that is, everyone. Drug companies deserve their just profits, but today far more money goes to marketing than to research, and we can live with less marketing.

Non-drug alternatives can save you even more money. Few of these alternatives have undergone rigorous study, whereas statins have been studied extensively. Furthermore, because of the lack of government regulation and standardization, supplements do not always contain the amounts claimed on their labels. My experience is that supplements from quality manufacturers with long track records are reliable. In addition, you can tell if a natural supplement is working when your cholesterol levels are checked. Thus, for many people, non-drug alternatives offer a reasonable, cost-effective alternative.

TABLE 11.3 CHOLESTEROL-LOWERING SUPPLEMENTS: COSTS AND COMPARISONS

Studies have shown that some supplements do not contain the amounts claimed on their labels. Therefore, I prefer using products from well-known companies with good quality control programs that produce pharmaceutical-grade products. However, if cost is an issue, you can start with a cheaper product and see if it lowers your cholesterol levels adequately.

PRODUCT	QUANTITY	COST/BOTTLE	MONTHLY COST
Red Yeast Rice			
Generic Internet Product 600 mg	45	$13	$17
Brand-Name Cholestin 600 mg	90	$63	$42
Policosanol			
Generic Internet Product 10 mg	90	$16	$11–$22
Pharmaceutical-Grade Co. 10 mg	60	$20	$20–$40
Plant Sterols (in comparison with prescription Zetia, which also blocks cholesterol absorption)			
Generic Plant Sterols 750 mg	60	$18	$18
Prescription Zetia 10 mg	90	$200	$67
Intermediate-Acting Niacin			
Prescription Niaspan 1,000 mg	100	$180	$60–$180
Inositol Hexaniacinate 500 mg	100	$20	$12–$36

CONCLUSION

Putting It All Together

For millions of people, the first symptom of heart disease will be a heart attack. Heart disease and strokes remain our number one and number three leading killers. Although these diseases may strike suddenly, they take decades to develop. You do not want to wait until they occur before getting serious about maintaining cardiovascular health. Atherosclerosis may be a slowly developing disease, but once entrenched it is difficult to stop and even more difficult to reverse.

An ounce of prevention is better than any amount of cure, because with cardiovascular disease, nothing matches prevention. Prevention begins with wise decisions made as early in life as possible. I would like to see every young person have a complete blood analysis that includes levels of cholesterol, C-reactive protein, triglycerides, homocysteine, small particle LDL, and lipoprotein A. Knowing where you stand is essential for knowing what to do.

Elevated cholesterol or CRP means prescription drugs for millions of people. We are a pill-oriented society, yet the most effective preventives and treatments for cardiovascular disease are a healthful diet, maintaining an ideal weight, exercising regularly, not smoking and, in my opinion, omega-3 oils from fish or supplements. With these, drug therapy for elevated cholesterol or CRP can often be avoided; if not avoided, doses can be minimized. Without these, cholesterol- and CRP-lowering drugs and supplements aren't nearly as effective anyway. By themselves, statins reduce the risk of cardiovascular disease by only about 30 percent. You can increase that a lot if you are willing to make the effort.

For most people who require medication for elevated LDL-C or CRP, treatment usually is not an emergency. The initial goal of treatment is not to reduce

LDL-C or other factors precipitously, but to start treatment in a way that is agreeable and comfortable for you. If you are like most people, you will not be happy to learn that you have a high LDL-C or CRP, and you will be stressed about having to make some tough adjustments in your lifestyle and perhaps about needing statin therapy for the rest of your life. Getting hit with unpleasant side effects is the last thing you need. It is well proven that people who remain in treatment after one year are very likely to remain long-term, so for most people the first goal of treatment should be to facilitate a successful beginning rather than forcing drastic cholesterol reduction instantly.

Treating elevated cholesterol or other factors is a marathon, not a sprint. There usually is time to get used to the idea that you have a medical condition and for you to begin making lifestyle changes. There is time to consider the various treatments and, whichever you choose, to use a start-low go-slow approach to guarantee that you get the right amount and nothing more. This means not over-doing it with drugs. This means not starting with higher doses than necessary.

As I have explained to doctors, FDA officials, and drug company executives, most people do not like taking medication. They hate the idea of needing drugs, especially drugs they have to take for the rest of their lives. If they must take medication, they want to take as little as possible. And if given a choice, most people opt for a start-low go-slow approach, because it is the only method that guarantees they will get the right amount of medication for them and nothing more. A start-low go-slow approach does not apply to every medication. Drugs like antibiotics, antifungals, and anti-cancer therapies must be strong enough to defeat these foreign or aberrant invaders. However, with the drugs that specifically target human systems, including the great majority of top-selling drugs such as statins, a precision-prescribing, start-low go-slow method makes sense. This method also applies to alternative therapies for reducing cardiac risk. Of course, before starting treatment, your doctor should make sure that other conditions are not causing your elevated cholesterol or CRP—medical conditions such as underactive thyroid, autoimmune disease, recent infection; drugs such as steroids or progestins; or supplements such as glucosamine, according to a few reports.

STATIN SENSE

Statin drugs—Lipitor, Zocor, Pravachol, Mevacor, Lescol—help millions upon millions of people. Statins lower LDL-C, raise HDL-C, reduce arterial inflammation and CRP, and inhibit atherosclerosis. When taken regularly, statins reduce heart attacks, strokes, and cardiovascular deaths. However, statin drugs can cause vexing side effects like muscle pain or abdominal discomfort. Some statin side effects are serious: liver injury, cognitive impairments, muscle degeneration, or kidney injury. Statin side effects are a main reason that 60 percent to 75 percent of people starting statins quit treatment.[1,2] Thus, although many doctors are enamored of statins, patients are not so sanguine. Many patients get side effects and little help from their doctors. Because of so many reported problems, in January 2004 *The Wall Street Journal* listed a backlash against statins as one of the ten most likely medical events in the coming year.[3] A backlash is not inevitable but will certainly occur if doctors and the drug industry don't improve their methods.

Stonewalling will not solve the problem. Dealing with the problem will, and it can be done quite simply. All of these side effects are dose-related, so the key to successful statin therapy is to make sure that you get the lowest dose you need. Many people need strong statin doses, but as many as 40 percent get better than average LDL-C reductions with statins and warrant low-dose therapy. What statin dose is right for you? That's impossible to predict, so the best way to tell is to start low and, if this isn't enough, increase gradually until the proper dose is achieved. In other words, start-low go-slow. *It does not matter whether you need a low dose, a high dose, or something in between—what matters is that you get the right statin dose for you and nothing more.* This is also important because long-term side effects with statins have now been discovered, and these side effects are directly correlated with the amount taken.

The precision-prescribing method is the best way to ensure that you get the right statin at the right dose for you. Precision-prescribing prevents excessive dosing and unnecessary side effects. This approach is particularly useful for people with moderate cholesterol elevations, as well as for at-risk groups such as seniors, women, people taking other medications, and medication-sensitive individuals. For these individuals, as well as for any person who simply wants to minimize the risks, the drug-company recommended initial statin doses are often unnecessarily strong.

Lower statin doses have been proven effective in study after study. Unfortunately, most doctors have never seen these studies and have no idea that low-dose statins can be very effective. Doctors assume that the drug companies and FDA have provided them with the lowest, safest doses. I assumed the same thing until I started looking into the side-effect problem and discovered otherwise. That is why I've compiled all of the current evidence in this book, so that you and your doctor can be informed about all of the possibilities before deciding on treatment.

What about people who require aggressive cholesterol-lowering therapy? Indeed, many people do, and the new guidelines issued by the American Heart Association in July 2004 make it clear that for people with acute or severe coronary artery disease, aggressive statin therapy is preferable. Still, it is important to match statin doses with these individuals, too. Aggressive treatment does not always have to start aggressively. Just because you may need aggressive statin therapy, this doesn't necessarily mean that your body is ready for super-strong statin doses from the start. High statin doses may reduce cholesterol and CRP levels more quickly, but they will also trigger many more side effects. Again, an individualized approach is the key.

Which statin should you use? When aggressive therapy is needed, many doctors prefer Lipitor or Zocor, but high doses of Pravachol and Mevacor may also do. Crestor is the most potent statin, but it should be used only for people who do not respond adequately to other statins. Crestor has the briefest track record and has already been linked to serious side effects. Some HMOs and insurers are switching to Mevacor because it is now available as generic lovastatin. Mevacor also has the longest track record of any statin and comes in a wide range of doses.

For mild-to-moderate cholesterol or CRP elevations, milder statins such as Pravachol, Mevacor, or Lescol are usually fine. Low doses of Zocor (5 or 10 mg) or splitting a 10-mg Lipitor tablet in half or in quarters also works. Some doctors employ full doses every other day.

Many alternative doctors strongly recommend coenzyme Q_{10} for anyone taking statins. This is particularly important for people experiencing muscle pain with statins.

ALTERNATIVE THERAPIES

Studies on the alternative therapies discussed in this book are relatively few in comparison with the hundreds of studies on statins. Yet the studies that exist on alternative therapies are generally favorable, and clinical experience supports these findings.

Red yeast rice and long-acting niacin (inositol nicotinate or hexaniacinate) are the most effective cholesterol-lowering alternative therapies. Because they cause few side effects and cost considerably less than prescription drugs, they are reasonable choices for people with mild-to-moderate cholesterol elevations and few risk factors. Red yeast rice, which contains a variety of natural statin-like substances, can also reduce CRP, as prescription statins do. Red yeast rice is not FDA approved for reducing cholesterol, mainly because the FDA monitors only the safety, not the effectiveness, of natural supplements.

There are many studies proving niacin's benefits. Mainstream doctors prefer time-released niacin preparations such as FDA-approved Niaspan, Niacor, or generic equivalents. Many alternative doctors prefer inositol hexaniacinate (hexanicotinate, nicotinate). Inositol hexaniacinate is not FDA approved, and there is some question about whether it works by releasing niacin itself or by some other mechanism. Nonetheless, inositol hexaniacinate seems to work and may cause fewer side effects, especially the flush or itching seen with Niaspan or similar products. And inositol hexaniacinate is inexpensive.

Policosanol, when derived from sugar cane, is effective for lowering LDL-C and triglycerides, and especially useful for elevating HDL-C. Plant sterols and soluble fiber (psyllium, pectin, oats and other foods) block cholesterol absorption and may be useful for modest cholesterol reductions or as adjuncts to other drug or alternative therapies. Fiber is known to reduce cholesterol levels. Garlic and soy have modest cholesterol-lowering effects.

The major drawback to non-drug alternatives is that the manufacturing is not regulated, and studies have shown that some supplement products do not contain the amounts claimed on the labels. For example, in a study published in the *Archives of Internal Medicine,* twenty-eight of fifty-nine preparations (47 percent) of the herb echinacea did not contain the amounts listed on the labels, and six preparations (10 percent) contained no echinacea at all. Products that claimed to be standardized were no more reliable than others.[4] However, manufacturing practices are improving in the nutriceutical industry, and many companies are having their products evaluated and standardized according to pharmaceutical standards by independent laboratories. I advise people to buy supplements made by reputable companies with long track records. Your alternative doctor can also recommend products with which he or she has obtained good results. Also, by monitoring your cholesterol or CRP levels, it should be apparent whether the supplement is working. It may be cheaper to buy bargain supplements, but getting effective treatment is far more important than saving a few pennies a day. Whether online or in a health food store, stick with products from well-known, reputable companies.

ESSENTIAL NUTRIENTS

Heart-healthy nutrients are very important. Omega-3 and omega-6 oils together lower LDL-C and raise HDL-C. Omega-3 oils reduce triglyceride levels. Most importantly, omega-3 oils produce a 45 percent to 80 percent reduction in the occurrence of sudden cardiac death, which causes 250,000 deaths annually.

Folic acid is important for reducing homocysteine, elevations of which are directly linked to cardiovascular disease. Magnesium promotes normal vascular functioning and reduces blood pressure and cardiac arrythmias. Coenzyme Q_{10} is essential for proper cell functioning and heart health, and may reduce muscle aches with statins.

Omega-3 oils, folic acid, CoQ_{10}, and magnesium are not supplements—they are nutrients that people need. Studies show that the great majority of Americans are deficient in omega-3 oils and magnesium, and these deficiencies undoubtedly play a role in the high incidence of high blood pressure, cardiac arrythmias, and sudden cardiac deaths. The fact that so many mainstream doctors do not know anything about these essential nutrients and do not discuss them with patients is deplorable and an example of the dominant drug-first mentality in mainstream medicine.

HEART-HEALTHY NUTRITION—YOUR BEST PREVENTATIVE

A heart attack or stroke is the culmination of thirty years of arterial injury. Cultures with diets based on vegetables, fruit, grains, and legumes rarely develop atherosclerosis or epidemics of coronary heart disease. They also have lower incidences of cancer. Good nutrition is the most effective preventive. Most people with high cholesterol do not have a medical disorder—they have a nutritional imbalance. Some people just cannot handle the saturated and hydrogenated fats so rife in our foods. Others cannot handle the ubiquitous sugars and refined grains. If you identify your weak link, fats or carbohydrates, and change your diet accordingly, suddenly you may not have high cholesterol or high blood pressure or diabetes anymore, and you may not need pill therapy.

Besides, taking pills does not erase all risks. Although a statin may reduce your cholesterol levels, the risk of cardiac disease is not entirely eliminated. Statins reduce cardiac risk about 30 percent. That isn't bad, but statins are not panaceas. This is why all experts stress prevention and why mainstream and alternative experts agree that a good diet, coupled with weight control and exercise, are the cornerstones of cardiovascular health.

Indeed, a recent study published in *JAMA* showed that diet can be as effective as statins in reducing LDL-cholesterol. In this controlled study, people eating a low-fat diet with cholesterol-lowering foods such as oat bran and cereal, soy drinks and foods, roasted almonds, and margarine containing plant sterols reduced LDL-C levels 29 percent. Another group taking 20 mg of lovastatin obtained LDL-C reductions of 31 percent—virtually the same. Both approaches also reduced C-reactive protein significantly.[5]

"I am not into statin bashing; heart disease is real and these drugs are saving lives every day," lead author of the study, Dr. David Jenkins of the University of Toronto's Department of Nutritional Sciences Faculty of Medicine, told UPI Science. "What I want to do is simply raise the question, again and again, of what should be the initial therapeutic approach to high LDL-cholesterol for anyone. This study confirms that the answer is, simply, a change in diet."[6]

"Managing diet is the key to treating all common lipid disorders," Dr. James Anderson, professor of medicine and clinical nutrition at the University of Kentucky in Lexington, stated in an accompanying editorial. "These results are potentially important, given the expense, safety concerns, and intolerance related to statin use."[7]

Unfortunately, this study, like others preceding it, is not likely to change our market-driven, advertising-shaped culture that pushes sugar-, fat-, and salt-laden foods that cause cardiovascular disease, then pushes expensive prescription drugs to slow (but not reverse) the damage. Our economic system is all about sales, not health. It is about profits, not prevention, and you are the cash cow. You can opt out by adopting a heart-healthy diet, exercising regularly, and keeping your weight down. With just 30–45 minutes of moderate exercise a day you can get almost all of the benefits of marathon training.

YOUR RIGHT OF INFORMED CONSENT: GETTING THE INFORMATION YOU NEED TO OBTAIN OPTIMAL MEDICAL TREATMENT

The physician has an ethical obligation to help the patient make choices from among the therapeutic alternatives consistent with good medical practice.[8]
> —AMERICAN MEDICAL ASSOCIATION CODE OF
> MEDICAL ETHICS

Using statins to reduce LDL-C and CRP is certainly consistent with "good medical practice," but so are the alternatives discussed in this book. Your doctor has an ethical obligation to inform you about all of these options, including "the therapeutic alternatives" that are proven effective. A doctor who doesn't is not fulfilling his or her obligation to provide you with sufficient information to exercise your right of informed consent. Before surgery, you are provided with a great deal of information to ensure that you receive informed consent. Indeed, you must sign a statement saying so. Informed consent applies as much to medication treatment as it does to surgery, yet fewer than 10 percent of patients ever receive fully informed consent when doctors prescribe drugs.

The AMA Code of Medical Ethics further states:

> The patient's right of self-decision can be effectively exercised only if the patient possesses enough information to enable an intelligent choice.[8]

Informed consent means, therefore, that you are entitled to enough information to make an intelligent choice about your own treatment. You cannot make an intelligent choice about statin therapy unless your doctor informs you about the lowest effective doses. You cannot make an intelligent choice about reducing cholesterol or other risk factors unless the treatment options include alternatives such as red yeast rice, niacin and inositol nicotinate, plant sterols, policosanol, and others. And in any plan to prevent or treat cardiovascular disease, you have a right to know about fish oils, folic acid, magnesium, and coenzyme Q_{10}.

Unfortunately, most doctors know little about these options and have scant time to learn. This is not an excuse, but a reality of today's mainstream medicine. You can help. Give your doctor a copy of this information. Help spread the word. Your doctor is not going to hear about effective non-drug alternatives from drug company sales reps, drug advertising, drug company–designed studies published in medical journals, or drug company-subsidized seminars and meetings. Doctors have so little time today, and there is so much information coming at them from so many different directions, you must take an active role in helping to keep your doctors current about the issues and options that concern you. Otherwise, most doctors will remain unaware of the solid data on low-dose statins or about how the precision-prescribing method can lower costs and reduce risks for patients.

Today, medical care is irrationally divided between two camps, mainstream and alternative. Mainstream medicine is overly reliant on pharmaceuticals as first-choice treatments, because doctors are trained to respect scientific studies. Most studies are conducted by the pharmaceutical industry or conducted at medical schools by researchers paid by drug companies to carry out studies underwritten and often designed by the companies. Many biases have been identified in drug company studies, which explains why they are 3.6 times more likely to be favorable than studies by independent researchers, yet the sheer mass of drug company studies published in medical journals influences doctors, especially when coupled with the influence of the drug industry within medical schools and the $15,000 spent by the drug industry on marketing directly to each doctor each year. The result is that, too often, medical decisions are based not on what is best for patients, but on what is marketed to doctors. Classic examples include doctors' writing millions of prescriptions for the synthetic hormones in Premarin and Prempro while ignoring natural, human-compatible hormones. Another example is that today doctors are prescribing Crestor to millions of people when much better known statins would work just as well.

Supplement manufacturers have little money to conduct studies or to send sales reps with armfuls of samples or to pay doctors to attend presentations. Patients' experiences and anecdotal reports may abound, but mainstream doctors are taught to be leery of such information and to believe nothing until it is proven in a double-blind, placebo-controlled study. Pharmaceuticals may be more expensive and more toxic than natural alternatives, but pharmaceutical companies have the money to conduct such studies, so this is where mainstream doctors turn. Of course, it is irrational to believe drug company information over the observations a doctor can make with his or her own patients, but this is what is happening, and it explains why drugs have become so dominant.

In a rational healthcare system, solutions for most disorders would begin with nutrition, then natural interventions, and then pharmaceuticals. The problem is, in today's medical-pharmaceutical complex where pharmaceutical companies have near total financial and informational control, and where doctors are taught to trust pharmaceuticals above all else, drugs are usually the first solution rather than the last. Even when we discover a new underlying mechanism of a disease, the research money does not go to finding a nutritional or natural solution. The money goes to finding a patentable, profitable, prescription synthetic product. When the new drug receives FDA approval, the media jumps on board, headlines abound, intensive marketing toward doctors and consumers begins—and is it any wonder why we are a drug-oriented society?

In other words, we have an irrational system, a divided system. We have hundreds of thousands of mainstream doctors who know drugs, think drugs, and prescribe drugs and little else. We have a few thousand alternative doctors who offer alternative methods. In an ideal system, all doctors would be integrative doctors, combining the best of both worlds. You shouldn't have to go to two doctors to get one full picture. All doctors should be knowledgeable about the full range of therapies for elevated cholesterol and CRP, as well as for everything else they treat. But this is the exception rather than the rule today.

My books, articles and *MedicationSense.com* website are dedicated to bridging the information gap in medicine today. Quality healthcare means good decisions based on good information. My goal is to provide a broad range of evidence-based information on pharmaceuticals, nutriceuticals, and nutrition for you and your doctor. By possessing all of the relevant, reliable information, the benefits and risks of treatments can be weighed. Decisions can be truly informed. With good, complete information, the benefits of medical treatment can be maximized, the risks can be minimized, and the healthcare system can be the "health" oriented system it is meant to be.

APPENDICES

Appendix A

Dr. Cohen's Principles for Safe, Effective Medication Therapy*

1. The best dose of any medication is the least amount that works. More is not necessarily better with medications.

2. Individual variation with medications isn't the exception; it's the rule. One person's proper dose is another person's overdose and another person's undertreatment.

3. Most side effects and adverse drug interactions are dose-related. The problem usually isn't the drugs, but the doses.

4. Many factors in drug research lead to the marketing of doses that are too strong for millions of people. Most at risk: seniors, women, people who have multiple medical disorders or are taking multiple medications, medication-sensitive individuals.

5. Except in acute cases, the first goal of treatment is to initiate treatment successfully.

6. Even aggressive therapy doesn't always have to start aggressively.

7. Most side effects can be prevented. If not prevented, their severity can be greatly reduced.

8. Minor side effects can have major consequences if they cause people to quit vital treatment.

9. The *start-low, go-slow* approach is a medically proven, safety-first method that is adaptable to the treatment of many common conditions.

10. People have a right to know about lower, safer drug doses that work.

People have a right to know about non-drug alternatives that work. These rights are contained in the Code of Medical Ethics.

*These principles apply to many top-selling drugs including statins and other cholesterol-lowering drugs, antihistamines, antihypertensives, antidepressants, anti-anxiety drugs, anti-inflammatory drugs, gastrointestinal drugs, sleep medications, some hormones, and others. However, these principles do not apply to treating acute disorders or to drugs with which undertreatment could cause harm, such as anti-cancer drugs, antibiotics and other anti-infectives, immunosuppressive drugs, anti-seizure drugs, and others. Decisions about your specific drugs and doses should always be made by your medical doctor.

Appendix B
Summary of
Cholesterol-Lowering Therapies

PRESCRIPTION DRUGS

Statins:
  Crestor (rosuvastatin)
  Lescol (fluvastatin)
  Lipitor (atorvastin)
  Mevacor (lovastatin, also available as a generic)
  Pravachol (pravastatin)
  Zocor (simvastatin)

Combinations that include statins:
  Advicor (Mevacor and Niaspan)
  Vytorin (Zocor and Zetia)

Prescription Niacin Derivatives:
  Niaspan
  Niaco
  Generics

Cholesterol Absorption Inhibitors:
  Welchol (colesevelam)
  Zetia (ezetimibe)
  Cholestyramine*

Fibric Acid Derivative:
  Lopid (gemfibrozil)*

NONPRESCRIPTION ALTERNATIVES**

Red Yeast Rice
Inositol Hexaniacinate (nicotinate, hexanicotinate)

Policosanol
Plant Sterols
Fiber
Guggulipid
Garlic
Soy
Pantethine
Tocotrienols

ADJUNCTIVE THERAPIES**

Folic acid (reduces homocysteine levels)
Essential fatty acids (omega-6 and omega-3 oils)
Coenzyme Q_{10}
Magnesium

*Not discussed in this book

**Not FDA-approved for lowering cholesterol levels or treating cardiovascular diseases (exception: soy).

References

Introduction

1. Gilman, A.G., Rall, T.W., Nies, A.S., Taylor, P. *Goodman and Gilman's The Pharmacological Basis of Therapeutics*. New York: Pergammon Press, 1990 and 1996.

2. Jackevicius, C.A., Mamdani, M., Tu, J.V. "Adherence with statin therapy in elderly patients with and without acute coronary syndromes." *JAMA* 2002;288:462–467.

3. Benner, J.S., Glynn, R.J., Mogun, H., et al. "Long-term persistence in use of statin therapy in elderly patients." *JAMA* 2002;288:455–461.

4. Ibid.

5. Wierzbicki, A.S., Lumb, P.J., Semra, et al. "Atorvastatin compared with simvastatin-based therapies in the management of severe familial hyperlipidaemias." *QJM* 1999;92(7):387–394.

6. Nawrocki, J.W., Weiss, S.R., Davidson, M.H., et al. "Reduction of LDL cholesterol by 25% to 60% in patients with primary hypercholesterolemia by atorvastatin, a new HMG-CoA reductase inhibitor." *Arteriosclerosis, Thrombosis, and Vascular Biology* 1995; 15(5):678–682.

7. Bertolini, S., et al. "Efficacy and safety of atorvastatin compared to pravastatin in patients with hypercholesterolemia." *Atherosclerosis* 1997;130(1–2):191–197.

8. Marz, W., et al. "Safety of low-density lipoprotein cholestrol reduction with atorvastatin versus simvastatin in a coronary heart disease population (the TARGET TANGIBLE trial)." *American Journal of Cardiology* 1999;84(1):7–13.

9. Lazarou, J., Pomeranz, B.H., Corey, P.N. "Incidence of adverse drug reactions in hospitalized patients: a meta-analysis of prospective studies." *JAMA* 1998;279(15): 1200–1205.

10. Braddock, C.H., Edwards, K.A., Hasenberg, N.M., Laidley, T.L., Levinson, W. "Informed Decision Making in Outpatient Practice: Time to Get Back to Basics." *JAMA* 1999;282:2313–2320.

Chapter 1

1. "Top 10 Drugs of 2001." *Pharmacy Times* 2002;68(4):10–15.

2. Noonan, D. "You want statins with that?" *Newsweek* 7/14/03:48–53.

3. Jackevicius, C.A., Mamdani, M., Tu, J.V. "Adherence with statin therapy in elderly patients with and without acute coronary syndromes." *JAMA* 2002;288:462–467.

4. Benner, J.S., Glynn, R.J., Mogun, H., et al. "Long-term persistence in use of statin therapy in elderly patients." *JAMA* 2002;288:455–461.

5. Cannon, C.P., Braunwald, E., McCabe, C.H., et al. "Comparison of intensive and moderate lipid lowering with statins after acute coronary syndromes." *The New England Journal of Medicine* 2004;350:1495–1504.

6. Nissen, S.E., Tuzcu, E.M., Schoenhagen, P., et al. "Effect of intensive compared with moderate lipid-lowering therapy on progression of coronary atherosclerosis: a randomized controlled trial." *JAMA* 2004;291:1071–1080.

7. Clark, W.G., Brater, D.C., Johnson, A.R. *Goth's Medical Pharmacology*, 13th edition. St. Louis: The C.V. Mosby Company, 1992.

8. American Society of Hospital Pharmacists. *American Hospital Formulary Service, Drug Information 2002*. Bethesda, MD: American Society of Hospital Pharmacists, 2002.

9. *Physicians' Desk Reference*, 54th–57th editions. Montvale, NJ: Medical Economics Company, 2000–2003.

10. Wierzbicki, A.S., Lumb, P.J., Semra, Y., et al. "Atorvastatin compared with simvastatin-based therapies in the management of severe familial hyperlipidaemias." *QJM* 1999;92(7):387–94.

11. Marz, W., Wollschlager, H., Klein, G., et al. "Safety of low-density lipoprotein cholestrol reduction with atorvastatin versus simvastatin in a coronary heart disease population (the TARGET TANGIBLE trial)." *American Journal of Cardiology* 1999;84(1):7–13.

12. Newman, C.B., Palmer, G., Silbershatz, H., Szarek, M. "Safety of atorvastatin derived from analysis of 44 completed trials in 9,416 patients." *American Journal of Cardiology* 2003;92(6):670–676.

13. Roberts, W.C. "The rule of 5 and the rule of 7 in lipid-lowering by statin drugs." *American Journal of Cardiology* 1997;80:106–107.

14. Bradford, R.H., Shear, C.L., Chremos, A.N., et al. "Expanded Clinical Evaluation of Lovastatin (EXCEL) study results. I. Efficacy in modifying plasma lipoproteins and adverse event profile in 8245 patients with moderate hypercholesterolemia." *Archives of Internal Medicine* 1991;151(1):43–49.

15. Pasternak, R.C., et al. "ACC/AHA/NHLBI Clinical Advisory on the Use and Safety of Statins." *Journal of the American College of Cardiology* 2002;40:567–572.

16. Lazarou, J., Pomeranz, B.H., Corey, P.N. "Incidence of adverse drug reactions in hospitalized patients: a meta-analysis of prospective studies" *JAMA* 1998;279(15):1200–1205.

17. Melmon, K.L., Morrelli, H.F., Hoffman, B.B., Nierenberg, D.W. *Melmon and Morrelli's Clinical Pharmacology: Basic Principles in Therapeutics*, 3rd edition. New York: McGraw-Hill, Inc., 1993.

18. American Medical Association. *AMA Drug Evaluations, Annual 1994*. Chicago: American Medical Association, 1994.

19. "Executive Summary of the Third Report of the National Cholesterol Education Program (NCEP) Expert Panel on Detection, Evaluation, and Treatment of High Blood Cholesterol in Adults (Adult Treatment Panel III)" *JAMA* 2001;285(19):2486–2497.

20. Cohen, J.S. *Over Dose: The Case Against The Drug Companies*. Tarcher/Putnam, New York: October 2001.

21. Parker-Pope, T. "Breakthrough! Ten major medical advances you're likely to see in the coming year." *The Wall Street Journal*, Jan. 26, 2004:R1.

22. Guideline for industry: Dose-response information to support drug registration. U.S. Food and Drug Administration, Nov. 1994, www.fda.gov/cder/guidance /iche4.pdf, accessed Feb. 22, 2003.

23. Gilman, A.G., Rall, T.W., Nies, A.S., Taylor, P. *Goodman and Gilman's The Pharmacological Basis of Therapeutics*. New York: Pergammon Press, 1990 and 1996.

24. Herxheimer, A. "Dosage needs systematic and critical review." *BMJ* 2001;323:253.

Chapter 2

1. Simopoulos, A.P., Robinson, J. *The Omega Diet*. New York: HarperCollins, 1999.

2. Roberts, W.C. "Getting more people on statins." *American Journal of Cardiology* 2002;9:683–685.

3. Whitaker, J. Treatments for Elevated Cholesterol. www.DrWhitaker.com:10/28/02.

4. Sacks, F.M., Pfeffer, M.A., Moye, L.A., et al. "The effect of pravastatin on coronary events after myocardial infarction in patients with average cholesterol levels. Cholesterol and Recurrent Events Trial investigators." *The New England Journal of Medicine* 1996; 335(14):1001–1009.

5. Shepherd, J., Cobbe, S.M., Ford, I., et al. "Prevention of coronary heart disease with pravastatin in men with hypercholesterolemia. West of Scotland Coronary Prevention Study Group." *The New England Journal of Medicine* 1995;333(20):1301–1307.

6. Downs, J.R., Clearfield, M., Weis, S., et al. "Primary prevention of acute coronary events with lovastatin in men and women with average cholesterol levels: results of AFCAPS/TexCAPS. Air Force/Texas Coronary Atherosclerosis Prevention Study." *JAMA* 1998;279(20):1615–1622.

7. "Randomised trial of cholesterol lowering in 4444 patients with coronary heart disease: the Scandinavian Simvastatin Survival Study(4S)." *Lancet* 1994;344(8934): 1383–1389.

8. The Long-Term Intervention with Pravastatin in Ischemic Disease (LIPID) Study Group. "Prevention of cardiovascular events and death with pravastatin in patients with coronary heart disease and a broad range of initial cholesterol levels." *The New England Journal of Medicine* 1998;339:1349–1357.

9. Gotto, A.M. Jr. "Lipid management in patients at moderate risk for coronary heart disease: insights from the Air Force/Texas Coronary Atherosclerosis Prevention Study (AFCAPS/TexCAPS)." *American Journal of Medicine* 1999;107(2A):36S–39S.

10. Executive Summary of the Third Report of the National Cholesterol Education Program (NCEP) Expert Panel on Detection, Evaluation, and Treatment of High Blood Cholesterol in Adults. *JAMA* 2001;285(19):2486–2497.

11. Jacotot, B., Banga, J.D., Pfister, P., Mehra, M. "Efficacy of a low dose-range of fluvastatin in the treatment of primary hypercholesterolaemia." *British Journal of Clinical Pharmacology* 1994;38(3):257–263.

12. Gonzalez, E.R. "The pharmacist's role in lipid reduction therapy." *Pharmacy Times* 63(4):65–70.

13. American Society of Hospital Pharmacists. *American Hospital Formulary Service, Drug Information 2002.* Gerald K. McEvoy, Editor. Bethesda, MD: American Society of Hospital Pharmacists, 2002.

14. Law, M.L., Watt, H.C., Wald, N.J. "The underlying risk of death after myocardial infarction in the absence of treatment." *Archives of Internal Medicine* 2002;162:2405–2410.

15. Cannon, C.P., Braunwald, E., McCabe, C.H., et al. "Comparison of intensive and moderate lipid lowering with statins after acute coronary syndromes." *The New England Journal of Medicine* 2004;350:1495–1504.

16. Ridker, P.M., Rifai, N., Rose, L., et al. R. "Comparison of C-reactive protein and low-density lipoprotein cholesterol levels in the prediction of first cardiovascular events." *The New England Journal of Medicine* 2002;347:1557–1565.

17. Albert, M.A., Glynn, R.J., Ridker, P.M. "Plasma concentration of C-reactive protein and the calculated Framingham Coronary Heart Disease Risk Score." *Circulation* 2003;108(2): 161–5.

18. Sinatra, S. "Statins: grossly overprescribed for cholesterol and underprescribed for internal inflammation." *The Sinatra Health Report*, Sept. 2002;8:1.

19. Grady, D. "Study Says a Protein May Be Better Than Cholesterol in Predicting Heart Disease Risk." *The New York Times;* NYTimes.com:Nov. 14, 2002.

20. Ravnskov, U. "Is atherosclerosis caused by high cholesterol?" *QJM* 2002;95:397–403.

21. Winslow, R. "Study Confirms Better Predictor of Heart Risk." *The Wall Street Journal,* Nov. 14, 2002:B1,3.

22. Walsh, B.W., Paul, S., Wild R.A., et al. "The Effects of Hormone Replacement Therapy and Raloxifene on C-Reactive Protein and Homocysteine in Healthy Postmenopausal Women: A Randomized, Controlled Trial." *Journal of Clinical Endocrinology and Metabolism* 2004;85:214–218.

23. Simopoulos, A.P. "Essential Fatty Acids in Health and Chronic Disease." *American Journal of Clinical Nutrition* 1999;70(suppl):560S–569S.

24. Simopoulos, A.P. "The Mediterranean diets: What is so special about the diet of Greece?" *Journal of Nutrition* 2001;131:3065S–3073S.

25. Block, G., Jensen, C., Dietrich, M., et al. "Plasma C-reactive protein concentrations in active and passive smokers: influence of antioxidant supplementation." *Journal of the American College of Nutrition* 2004;23:141–147.

26. Ariyo, A.A., Thach, C., Tracy, R. "Lp(a) Lipoprotein, Vascular Disease, and Mortality in the Elderly." *The New England Journal of Medicine* 2003;349:2108–2115.

27. Saely, C.H., Marte, T., Drexel, H. "Lp(a) Lipoprotein, Vascular Disease, and Mortality in the Elderly." *The New England Journal of Medicine* 2004;350:1150–1152.

28. Ehmke, J. More reasons to avoid statin drugs: does Lipitor raise lipoprotein A? Dr. Mercola Website, Aug. 13, 2003:www.mercola.com/2003/aug/13/statin_drugs.htm.

29. McCully, K.S. "Homocysteine, folate, vitamin B6, and cardiovascular disease." *JAMA* 1998;280:417.

30. Fager, G., Wiklund, O. "Cholesterol reduction and clinical benefit. Are there limits to our expectations?" *Arteriosclerosis, Thrombosis, and Vascular Biology,* 1997;17(12):3527–3533.

31. Lewis, S.J., Moye, L.A., Sacks, F.M., et al. "Effect of pravastatin on cardiovascular events in older patients with myocardial infarction and cholesterol levels in the average range. Results of the Cholesterol and Recurrent Events (CARE) trial." *Annals of Internal Medicine* 1998;129(9):681–689.

32. "West of Scotland Coronary Prevention Study: identification of high-risk groups and comparison with other cardiovascular intervention trials." *Lancet* 1996;348(9038):1339–1342.

33. Moriarty, P.M. "Using Both "relative risk reduction" and "number needed to treat" in evaluating primary and secondary clinical trials of lipid reduction." *American Journal of Cardiology,* 2001;87(10):1206.

34. Therapeutics Initiative of the University of British Columbia. "Do Statins have a role in primary prevention?" *Therapeutics Letter* 2004;48:www.ti.ubc.ca/pages/letter48.htm.

35. Corvol, J., Bouzamondo, A., Sirol, M., et al. "Differential effects of lipid-lowering therapies on stroke prevention." *Archives of Internal Medicine* 2003;163:669–676.

36. Grundy, S.M., Cleeman, J.I., Bairey, C.N., et al. "Implications of recent clinical trials for the National Cholesterol Education Program Adult Treatment Panel III Guidelines." *Circulation* 2004;110:227–239.

Chapter 3

1. Zuger, A. "Caution: That dose may be too high." *The New York Times,* September 17, 2002:nytimes.com.

2. Cohen, J.S. *Over Dose: The Case Against The Drug Companies.* Tarcher/Putnam, New York: October 2001.

3. Cohen, J.S. "Do standard doses of frequently prescribed drugs cause preventable adverse effects in women?" *JAMWA (The Journal of the American Medical Women's Association)* 2002;57:105–110.

4. Cohen, J.S. "Dose discrepancies between the Physicians' Desk Reference and the medical literature, and their possible role in the high incidence of dose-related adverse drug events." *Archives of Internal Medicine* April 9, 2001:161:957–964.

5. Cohen, J.S. "Adverse drug effects, compliance, and the initial doses of antihypertensive drugs recommended by the Joint National Committee vs. the Physicians' Desk Reference." *Archives of Internal Medicine* March 26, 2001;161:880–885.

6. Cohen, J.S. "Ways to minimize adverse drug reactions: individualized doses and common sense are key." *Postgraduate Medicine* 1999;106:163–172.

7. Cohen J.S., Insel P.A. "The Physicians' Desk Reference. Problems and possible improvements." *Archives of Internal Medicine* 1996;156(13):1375–1380.

8. Peck, C.C. "Drug development: improving the process." *Food Drug Law Journal* 1997;52:163–167.

9. Herxheimer, A. "How much drug in the tablet?" *Lancet* 1991;337:346–348.

10. Frolkis, J.P., Pearce, G.L., Nambi, V. "Statins do not meet expectations for lowering low-density lipoprotein cholesterol levels when used in clinical practice." *American Journal of Medicine* 2002;113:625–629.

11. Pfizer Inc. Lipitor advertisement. *Postgraduate Medicine* 2000;7:47.

12. Ehrlich, R. The lower dose alternative. *DTC in Perspective*, Newsletter for DTC Executives, Jan. 18, 2002;9: website.

13. U.S. Food and Drug Administration. CDER 2002 Report to the Nation: Improving Public Health through Human Drugs. Rockville, MD 20857, www.fda.gov, accessed 6/3/04.

14. Steinhagen-Thiessen, E. "Comparative efficacy and tolerability of 5 and 10 mg simvastatin and 10 mg pravastatin in moderate primary hypercholesterolemia. Simvastatin Pravastatin European Study Group." *Cardiology* 1994;85(3–4):244–254.

15. Tuomilehto, J., Guimaraes, A.C., Kettner, et al. "Dose-response of simvastatin in primary hypercholesterolemia." *Journal of Cardiovascular Pharmacology* 1994;24(6):941–949.

16. Bristol-Myers Squibb. Advisory Committee Meeting Briefing Book for the Rx to OTC Switch of Pravachol (Pravastatin Sodium). Joint Meeting of Nonprescription Drugs Advisory Committee and Endocrinologic and Metabolic Drugs Advisory Committee, FDA website, June 2000:www.fda.gov/ohrms/dockets/ac/00/backgrd/3622b2a_part1.pdf, accessed July 2001.

17. Nonprescription Mevacor, FDA Advisory Committee Background Information, FDA Website, June 2000:www.fda.gov/ohrms/dockets/ac/00/backgrd/3622b1b.pdf, accessed July 2001.

18. Smith, D.L. *DTC Perspectives* Jan.-Feb. 2002;1(2):52–56.

19. Barsky, A., Saintfort, R., et al. "Nonspecific medication side effects and the nocebo phenomena." *JAMA* 2002;287:622–627.

20. Grundy, S.M., Cleeman, J.I., Bairey, C.N., et al. "Implications of recent clinical trials for the National Cholesterol Education Program Adult Treatment Panel III Guidelines." *Circulation* 2004;110:227–239.

21. Stolberg, S.G., Gerth, J. "How research benefits marketing." *The New York Times*, Dec. 23, 2000:www.nytimes.com.

22. Sinatra, S. "The Cholesterol Myth." *The Sinatra Health Report*, June 12, 2003.

23. More Crestor Safety Concern; Call for Ban Renewed. *Dickinson's FDA Webview*, 5/17/2004, www.fdaweb.com.

24. Wolfe, S.M. "Updates: rosuvastatin (Crestor) and nefazodone (Serzone) continue as do not use drugs." *Worst Pills, Best Pills News*, Apr. 2004;10:28–29.

25. Wolfe, S.M. "Further reasons why the cholesterol-lowering "statin" drug rosuvastatin (Crestor) is a do not use drug." *Worst Pills, Best Pills News*, March 2004;10:17–19.

26. Horton, R. "The statin wars: why AstraZeneca must retreat [editorial]." *Lancet* 2003 (Oct. 25);362:1341.

27. Parker-Pope, T. "Applying pressure: government takes on drug makers over treating hypertension." *The Wall Street Journal*, Feb. 17, 2004:D1.

28. Harris, G. "FDA Failing in Drug Safety, Officer Asserts." *The New York Times*, Nov. 19, 2004, www.nytimes.com.

Chapter 4

1. Frolkis, J.P., Pearce, G.L., Nambi, V. "Statins do not meet expectations for lowering low-density lipoprotein cholesterol levels when used in clinical practice." *American Journal of Medicine* 2002;113:625–629.

2. Cohen, J.S. "Dose discrepancies between the Physicians' Desk Reference and the medical literature, and their possible role in the high incidence of dose-related adverse drug events." *Archives of Internal Medicine*, April 9, 2001:161:957–964.

3. Food and Drug Administration. Guideline for industry: Dose-response information to support drug registration. U.S. Food and Drug Administration, www.fda.gov/cder/guidance/iche4.pdf:Nov. 1994; accessed Feb. 22, 2003.

4. *Physicians' Desk Reference*, 54th-57th Editions. Montvale, NJ: Medical Economics Company, 2000–2003.

5. Nowrocki, J., Weiss, S., et al. "Reduction in LDL cholesterol by 25% to 60% in patients with primary hypercholesterolemia by atorvastatin, a new HMG-Co-A reductase inhibitor." *Arteriosclerosis, Thrombosis, and Vascular Biology* 1995;15:678–682.

6. Wolffenbuttel, B.H., Mahla, G., Muller, D., et al. "Efficacy and safety of a new cholesterol synthesis inhibitor, atorvastatin, in comparison with simvastatin and pravastatin, in subjects with hypercholesterolemia." *Netherlands Journal of Medicine* 1998;52(4):131–137.

7. Bakker-Arkema, R.G., Davidson, M.H., Goldstein, R.J., et al. "Efficacy and safety of a new HMG-CoA reductase inhibitor, atorvastatin, in patients with hypertriglyceridemia." *JAMA* 1996;275(2):128–133.

8. Bakker-Arkema, R.G., Best, J., Fayyad, R., et al. "A brief review paper of the efficacy and safety of atorvastatin in early clinical trials." *Atherosclerosis* 1997;131(1):17–23.

9. Cilla, D.D. Jr., Whitfield, L.R., Gibson, D.M., et al. "Multiple-dose pharmacokinetics, pharmacodynamics, and safety of atorvastatin, an inhibitor of HMG-CoA reductase, in healthy subjects." *Clinical Pharmacology and Therapeutics* 1996;60(6):687–695.

10. Steinhagen-Thiessen. E. "Comparative efficacy and tolerability of 5 and 10 mg simvastatin and 10 mg pravastatin in moderate primary hypercholesterolemia. Simvastatin Pravastatin European Study Group." *Cardiology* 1994;85(3–4):244–254.

11. Tuomilehto, J., Guimaraes, A.C., Kettner, H., et al. "Dose-response of simvastatin in primary hypercholesterolemia." *Journal of Cardiovascular Pharmacology* 1994;24(6):941–949.

12. Hunninghake, D., Bakker-Arkema, R.G., Wigand, J.P., et al. "Treating to meet NCEP-recommended LDL cholesterol concentrations with atorvastatin, fluvastatin, lovastatin, or simvastatin in patients with risk factors for coronary heart disease." *Journal of Family Practice* 1998;47(5):349–356.

13. Bristol-Myers Squibb. Advisory Committee Meeting Briefing Book for the Rx to OTC Switch of Pravachol (Pravastatin Sodium). Joint Meeting of Nonprescription Drugs Advisory Committee and Endocrinologic and Metabolic Drugs Advisory Committee, FDA website, June 2000: www.fda.gov/ohrms/dockets/ac/00/backgrd/3622b2a_part1.pdf, accessed July 2001.

14. Jones, P.H., Farmer, J.A., Cressman, M.D., et al. "Once-daily pravastatin in patients with primary hypercholesterolemia: a dose-response study." *Clinical Cardiology* 1991;14(2):146–151.

15. Nonprescription Mevacor, FDA Advisory Committee Background Information, FDA Website, June 2000:www.fda.gov/ohrms/dockets/ac/00/backgrd/3622b1b.pdf, accessed July 2001.

16. Rubinstein, A., Lurie, Y., Groskop, I., et al. "Cholesterol-lowering effects of a 10 mg daily dose of lovastatin in patients with initial total cholesterol levels 200 to 240 mg/dl(5.18 to 6.21 mmol/liter)." *American Journal of Cardiology* 1991;68(11):1123–1126.

17. Arca, M., Vega, G.L., Grundy, S.M. "Hypercholesterolemia in postmenopausal women: metabolic defects and response to low-dose lovastatin." *JAMA* 1994;271(6):453–459.

18. Crestor Package Insert. Wilmington DE: AstraZeneca Pharmaceuticals LP, 2003.

19. FDA "Case Studies" on Dosing Problems Include Lotronex, Crestor. "The Pink Sheet" on the Web, Nov. 24, 2003:65:24.

20. Olsson, A.G., Pears, J., McKellar, J., et al. "Effect of rosuvastatin on low-density lipoprotein cholesterol in patients with hypercholesterolemia." *American Journal of Cardiology* 2001;88:504–508.

21. Olsson, A.G. "A new statin: a new standard." *The American Journal of Managed Care* 2001;7:S152.

22. Iliff, D. "Guidelines for diagnosis and treatment of high cholesterol (letter)." *JAMA* 2001;286:2402–2403.

23. Matalka, M.S., Ravnan, M.C., Deedwania, P.C. "Is alternate daily dose of atorvastatin effective in treating patients with hyperlipidemia? The Alternate Day Versus Daily Dosing of Atorvastatin Study." *American Heart Journal* 2002;144:674–677.

24. Brown, B.G., et al. "Simvastatin and niacin, antioxidant vitamins, or the combination for the prevention of coronary disease." *The New England Journal of Medicine* 2001;345(22):1583–1591.

25. Sprecher D.L., Abrams J., Allen J.W., et al. "Low-dose combined therapy with fluvastatin and cholestyramine in hyperlipidemic patients." *Annals of Internal Medicine* 1994;120(7):537–543.

26. Chazerain, P., Hayem, G., Hamza, S., et al. "Four cases of tendinopathy in patients on statin therapy." *Journal of Joint, Bone, and Spine* 2001;68:430–433.

27. Pierson, R., Tobin, E. Merck Cautions about Use of Zocor with Heart Drug. *Reuters Company News*, June 6, 2002: website.

28. Moore, T.J., Psaty, B.M., Furberg, C.D. "Time to act on drug safety." *JAMA* 1998;279(19):1571–1573.

29. Moore, T.J. In short drug tests, fatal flaws: a narrow focus on effectiveness is a prescription for harm. *Boston Globe*, July 14, 2002:website.

30. Gaist, D., Jeppesen, U., Andersen, M., et al. "Statins and the risk of polyneuropathy: a case-control study." *Neurology* 2002;58:1333–1337.

31. "Peripheral neuropathy due to statins: a rare but potentially incapacitating adverse effect." *Prescribe International* 2000;9:115.

32. "Choice of lipid-lowering drugs." *The Medical Letter On Drugs And Therapeutics* 1996;38:67–69.

33. Whitaker, J. *The MD's Drug and Supplement Interaction Guide*. Potomac, MD: Phillips Health, 2002.

34. Sinatra, S. How to lower your cholesterol level. DrSinatra.com:3/3/O3.

35. Dickinson, J.G. "Statin warning urged to offset new Merck patents." *Dickinson's FDA Review*, June 2002;9:7–8.

36. Wolfe, S.M. "Do Not Use Until October 2009: Zetia (Ezetimibe) or Vytorin (Ezetimibe with Simvastatin) for Cholesterol Lowering." *Worst Pills, Best Pills News* Dec. 2004;10(12):89–92.

Chapter 5

1. Gilman, A.G., Rall, T.W., Nies, A.S., Taylor, P. *Goodman and Gilman's The Pharmacological Basis of Therapeutics*. New York: Pergammon Press, 1990 and 1996.

2. Weinshilbourn, R. "Inheritance and drug response." *The New England Journal of Med icine* 2003;348:529–537.

3. Sjoqvist, F., Bertilsson, L. "Clinical pharmacology of antidepressant drugs: Pharmacogenetics." *Advances in Biochemical Psychopharmacology* 1984;39:359–372.

4. Phillips, K.A., Veenstra, D.L., Oren, E., et al. "Potential role of pharmacogenomics in reducing adverse drug reactions: a systematic review." *JAMA* 2001;286:2270–2279.

5. Drug Interactions. *The Medical Letter On Drugs and Therapeutics* 2000;45:46–48.

6. Chasman, D.I., Posada, D., Subrahmanyan, L., et al. "Pharmacogenetic study of statin therapy and cholesterol reduction." *JAMA* 2004;291:2821–2827.

7. Genes play role in who benefits from statin: In boost to "personalized medicine," study links patient genetics with efficacy of cholesterol drug." *The Wall Street Journal*, June 16, 2004:D1.

8. Melmon, K.L., Morrelli, H.F., Hoffman, B.B., Nierenberg, D.W. *Melmon and Morrelli's Clinical Pharmacology: Basic Principles in Therapeutics*, 3rd edition. New York: McGraw-Hill, Inc., 1993.

9. *United States Pharmacopeia, Drug Information (USP DI)*: Drug Information for the Health Care Professional. Taunton, MA: Rand McNally, 1994.

Chapter 6

1. Welty, F.K. "Cardiovascular Disease and Dyslipidemia in Women." *Archives of Internal Medicine* 2001;161:514–522.

2. Simopoulos, A.P., Robinson, J. *The Omega Diet*. New York: HarperCollins, 1999.

3. Wierzbicki A.S., Lumb P.J., Chik G., Crook M.A. "High-density lipoprotein choles-terol and triglyceride response with simvastatin versus atorvastatin in familial hyper-cholesterolemia." *American Journal of Cardiology* 2000;86(5):547–549.

4. Cheng H., Rogers J.D., Sweany A.E., et al. "Influence of age and gender on the plas-ma profiles of 3-hydroxy-3-methylglutaryl-coenzyme A (HMG-CoA) reductase inhibitory activity following multiple doses of lovastatin and simvastatin." *Pharma-ceutical Research.* 1992;9:1629–1633.

5. Ose, L., Luurila, O., Eriksson, J., et al. "Efficacy and safety of cerivastatin, 0.2 mg and 0.4 mg, in patients with primary hypercholesterolaemia: A multinational, randomised, double-blind study. Cerivastatin Study Group." *Current Medical Research and Opinion* 1999;15:228–240.

6. Hendler, S. Scripps Clinic Conference on Evidence-Based Alternative Therapies. La Jolla, CA, Jan. 2004.

7. Pleym, H., Spigset, O., Kharasch, E.D., Dale, O. "Gender differences in drug effects: implications for anesthesiologists." *Acta Anesthesiologica Scandinavica* 2003;47:241–259.

8. Cohen, J.S. "Do standard doses of frequently prescribed drugs cause preventable adverse effects in women?" *JAMWA* 2002;57:105–110.

9. Thurmann, P.A., Hompesch, B.C. "Influence of gender on the pharmacokinetics and pharmacodynamics of drugs." *International Journal of Clinical Pharmacology and Thera-peutics* 1998;36(11):586–590.

10. Women Sufficiently Represented in New Drug Testing, but FDA Oversight Needs Improvement. Report to Congressional Requesters. US General Accounting Office, GAO-01–754, July 6, 2001:www.fda.gov/womens/informat.html.

11. Atkin, P.A., Sheffield, G.M. "Medication-related adverse reactions and the elderly: a literature review." *Adverse Drug Reactions and Toxicology Review* 1995;14:175–191.

12. "Exploring the Biological Contributions to Human Health: Does Sex Matter?" Wiz-emann, T.M., Pardue, M.L., Editors. Committee on Understanding the Biology of Sex and Gender Differences, Board on Health Sciences Policy, National Academy of Sci-ences, National Academy Press, 2001.

13. Kritz, F.L. "Mars and Venus and Drugs: Sex Differences Create Extra Risks for Women." *Washington Post,* Feb. 20, 2001:T7.

14. Roe, C.M., McNamara, A.M., Motheral, B.R. "Gender- and age-related prescription drug use patterns." *Pharmacoepidemiology* 2002;36:30–39.

15. Bowman, L. "51% Of U.S. Adults Take 2 Pills or More a Day, Survey Reports (Scripps Howard News Service)." *San Diego Union-Tribune,* Jan. 17, 2001:A8.

16. Jenkins, A.J. "Might money spent on statins be better spent (letter)?" *BMJ* 2003;327:933.

17. Smucker, W.D., Kontak, J.R. "Adverse drug reactions causing hospital admission in an elderly population: experience with a decision algorithm." *Journal of the American Board of Family Practice* 1990;3(2):105–109.

18. Montamat, S.C., Cusack, B.J., Vestal, R.E. "Management of drug therapy in the eld-erly." *The New England Journal of Medicine* 1989;321(5):303–309.

19. *Physicians' Desk Reference,* 54th edition. Montvale, NJ: Medical Economics Compa-ny, 2000.

20. Antonicelli, R., Onorato G., Pagelli P., et al. "Simvastatin in the treatment of hyper-cholesterolemia in elderly patients." *Clinical Therapeutics* 1990;12(2):165–171.

21. Chan, P., Lee, C.B., Lin, T.S., et al. "The effectiveness and safety of low dose pravas-tatin in elderly hypertensive hypercholesterolemic subjects on antihypertensive thera-py." *American Journal of Hypertension* 1995;8(11):1099–1104.

22. Lansberg, P.J., Mitchel, Y.B., Shapiro, D., et al. "Long-term efficacy and tolerability of simvastatin in a large cohort of elderly hypercholesterolemic patients." *Atheroscle-rosis* 1995;116(2):153–162.

23. Arca, M., Vega, G.L., Grundy, S.M. "Hypercholesterolemia in postmenopausal women: metabolic defects and response to low-dose lovastatin." *JAMA* 1994;271(6):453–459.

24. Williams, R.D. "Medications and older adults." *FDA Consumer Magazine,* Sept.-Oct. 1997.

25. Ariyo, A.A., Thach, C., Tracy, R. "Lp(a) lipoprotein, vascular disease, and mortali-ty in the elderly." *The New England Journal of Medicine* 2003;349:2108–2115.

26. Saely, C.H., Marte, T., Drexel, H. "Lp(a) lipoprotein, vascular disease, and mortali-ty in the elderly." *The New England Journal of Medicine* 2004;350:1150–1152.

27. Rochon, P.A., Anderson, G.M., Tu, J.V., et al. "Age- and gender-related use of low-dose drug therapy: the need to manufacture low-dose therapy and evaluate the mini-mum effective dose." *Journal of the American Geriatrics Society* 1999;47(8):954–959.

28. Clark, W.G., Brater, D.C., Johnson, A.R. *Goth's Medical Pharmacology,* 13th edition. St. Louis: The C.V. Mosby Company, 1992.

29. Wolfe, S.M., Hope, R.E. *Worst Pills, Best Pills II: The Older Adult's Guide to Avoiding Drug-Induced Death or Illness.* Washington, D.C.: Public Citizen's Health Research Group, 1993.

30. Everitt, D.E., Avorn, J. "Drug prescribing for the elderly." *Archives of Internal Medi-cine,* 1986;146(12):2393–2396.

31. Rochon, P.A., Gurwitz, J.H. "Optimising drug treatment for elderly people: the pre-scribing cascade." *BMJ* 1997;315(7115):1096–1099.

Chapter 7

1. Duerksen, S. "2 San Diego Scientists Raise Questions about Cholesterol-Cutting Drugs." *San Diego Union-Tribune,* May 28, 2001:A1,18.

2. Benner, J.S., et al. "Long-term persistence in use of statin therapy in elderly patients." *JAMA* 2002;288:455–461.

3. Avorn, J. "The prescription as final common pathway." *International Journal of Tech-nology Assessment in Health Care,* 1995:11(3):384–390.

4. Woosley, R.L. Personal communication, April 19, 2002.

5. Very Few Students in American Medical Schools Receive Training about Adverse Drug Events. U.S. Agency for Healthcare Research and Quality, U.S. Department of Health and Human Services, Sept. 4, 2001:www.ahcpr.gov/news/press/pr2001/studntpr.htm, accessed Apr. 9, 2003.

6. Gandhi, T.K., Burstin, H.R., Cook, E.F., et al. "Drug complications in outpatients." *Journal of General Internal Medicine* 2000;15:149–154.

7. Michels, K.B. "Problems assessing nonserious adverse drug reactions: antidepressant drug therapy and sexual dysfunction." *Pharmacotherapy* 1999;19(4):424–429.

8. Parker-Pope, T. "Health Matters: Cholesterol drugs may cause side effects that mimic aging." *The Wall Street Journal*, Dec. 16, 2002.

9. Herxheimer, A. "Possible harm from drugs: when and how to inform doctors and users." Talk given at the 7th annual meeting of the European Society of Pharmacovigilance, Ankara, 23 Sept 1999. *Médecine Légale Hospitaliére* 2000;3:49–50.

10. Brody, J.E. "Statins: Miracles for some, menace for a few." *The New York Times*, Dec. 10, 2002:nytimes.com.

11. Graedon, J., Graedon, T. Muscle pain may be side effect of cholesterol medications. *Los Angeles Times*, Dec. 8, 2003:website.

12. Sinatra, S. "Statins: grossly overprescribed for cholesterol and underprescribed for internal inflammation." *The Sinatra Health Report*, Sept. 2002;8:1.

13. Rochon, P.A., Gurwitz, J.H. "Optimising drug treatment for elderly people: the prescribing cascade." *BMJ* 1997;315(7115):1096–1099.

14. Gurwitz, J.H., Field, T.S. "Adverse Drug Effects in Ambulatory Elderly Patients-Reply." *JAMA* 2003;289:3238–3239.

15. Cimons, M. "Scientists Study Gender Gap in Drug Responses." *Los Angeles Times*, Sun. June 6, 1999: A-1,8–9.

16. Sheehan, D.V., Hartnett-Sheehan, K. "The role of SSRIs in panic disorder." *Journal of Clinical Psychiatry* 1996;517(10 suppl):51–58.

17. Graedon, J., Graedon, T. *Los Angeles Times*, Mon. May 21, 2000: S-2,6.

18. Parker-Pope, T. "Breakthrough! Ten major medical advances you're likely to see in the coming year." *The Wall Street Journal*, Jan. 26, 2004:R1.

19. Williams, J. "New research has changed physician's life." *San Diego Union-Tribune*, Feb. 16, 2004:C3.

20. Naranjo, C.A., Busto, U., Sellers, E.M., et al. "A method for estimating the probability of adverse drug reactions." *Clinical Pharmacology and Therapeutics* 1981;30:239–245.

21. Brodell, R.T. "Do more than discuss that unusual case." *Postgraduate Medicine* 2000;108:19–21.

22. Gitlin, M.J. "Effects of depression and antidepressants on sexual functioning." *Bulletin of the Menninger Clinic* 1995:59(2):232–248.

23. Hirschfeld, R.M. "Management of sexual side effects of antidepressant therapy." *Journal of Clinical Psychiatry* 1999;60(Suppl 14):27–30.

24. Montejo-Gonzalez, A.L., Llorca, G., Izquierdo, J.A., et al. "SSRI-induced sexual dysfunction: fluoxetine, paroxetine, sertraline, and fluvoxamine in a prospective, multi-center, and descriptive clinical study of 344 patients." *The Journal of Sex and Marital Therapy* 1997;23(3):176–194.

25. Kessler, D.A., Rose, J.L., Temple, R.J., Schapiro, R., Griffin, J.P. "Therapeutic-class

wars—drug promotion in a competitive marketplace." *New England Journal of Medicine* 1994;331(20):1350–1353.

26. Dickinson, J.G. "FDA OKs new drugs that over-dose millions, physician says; FDA replies." *Dickinson's FDA Review*, 2002;9(1):3,10–15.

27. Herxheimer, A. "Dosage needs systematic and critical review." *BMJ* 2001;323.

28. Executive Summary of the Third Report of the National Cholesterol Education Program (NCEP) Expert Panel on Detection, Evaluation, and Treatment of High Blood Cholesterol in Adults. *JAMA* 2001;285(19):2486–2497.

29. Gilman, A.G., Rall, T.W, Nies, A.S., Taylor, P. *Goodman and Gilman's The Pharmacological Basis of Therapeutics.* New York: Pergamon Press, 1990 and 1996.

30. Barnett, B.P. Department of Health and Human Services, Food and Drug Administration, Public Hearing on FDA Regulation of Over-the-Counter Products, June 29, 2000:151.

31. Hill, C., Zeitz, C., Kirkham, B. "Dermatomyositis with lung involvement in a patient treated with simvastatin." *Australian and New Zealand Journal of Medicine* 1995;25:745–746.

32. Sridhar, M.K., Abdulla, A. "Fatal lupus-like syndrome and ARDS induced by fluvastatin." *Lancet* 1998;352(9122):114.

33. de Groot, R.E.B., Willems, L.N.A., Dijkman, J.H. "Interstitial lung disease with pleural effusion caused by simvastin " *Journal of Internal Medicine* 1996;239:361 363.

34. Rosch, P. "Guidelines for diagnosis and treatment of high cholesterol (letter)." *JAMA* 2001;286:2400–2402.

35. *Physicians' Desk Reference*, 53rd-57th editions. Montvale, NJ: Medical Economics Company, 1999–2003.

36. Cohen, J.S. "Adverse drug effects, compliance, and the initial doses of antihypertensive drugs recommended by the Joint National Committee vs. the Physicians' Desk Reference." *Archives of Internal Medicine* 2001;161:880–885.

37. Cohen, J.S. *Make Your Medicine Safe: How To Prevent Side Effects From The Drugs You Take.* New York: Avon Books, 1998.

Chapter 8

1. Ault, A. "U.S. alternative medicine report spurs controversy." *Reuters Health,* Mar. 25, 2002:www.reuters.com.

2. Villarosa, L. "The verdict is still out on alternative medicine." *The New York Times,* Apr. 13, 2002:nytimes.com.

3. Heber, D., Lembertas, A., Qy, L., et al. "An analysis of nine proprietary Chinese red yeast rice dietary supplements." *Journal of Alternative and Complementary Medicine* 2001;7:133–139.

4. Morelli, V., Zoorob, R.J. "Congestive Heart Failure and Hypercholesterolemia: Alternative Therapies, Part 2." *American Family Physician* 2000;62:1325–1330.

5. Heber, D., Yip, I., Ashley, J.M., et al. "Cholesterol-lowering effects of a proprietary

Chinese red-yeast-rice dietary supplement." *American Journal of Clinical Nutrition* 1999;69:231–236.

6. Keithley, J.K., Swanson, B., Sha, B.E., et al. "A pilot study of the safety and efficacy of cholestin in treating HIV-related dyslipidemia." *Nutrition* 2002;18:201–204.

7. Patrick, L., Uzick, M. "Cardiovascular disease: C-reactive protein and the inflammatory disease paradigm." *Alternative Medicine Review* 2001;6:248–271.

8. Schardt, D. "The heart of the matter: some supplements work . . . , others are worthless." *Nutrition Action Health Letter* 2004;31:8–11.

9. Executive Summary of the Third Report of the National Cholesterol Education Program (NCEP) Expert Panel on Detection, Evaluation, and Treatment of High Blood Cholesterol in Adults. *JAMA* 2001;285(19):2486–2497.

10. Whitaker, J. *Slash Your Cholesterol in 30 Days without Drugs*. Potomac, MD: Phillips Health, 2002.

11. McKenney, J. "New perspectives on the use of niacin in the treatment of lipid disorders." *Archives of Internal Medicine* 2004;164:697–705.

12. American Society of Hospital Pharmacists. *American Hospital Formulary Service, Drug Information 2002*. Gerald K. McEvoy, editor. Bethesda, MD: American Society of Hospital Pharmacists: 2002.

13. *Physicians' Desk Reference*, 54th Edition. Montvale, NJ: Medical Economics Company, 2000.

14. Head, K.A. "Inositol hexaniacinate: a safer alternative to niacin." *Alternative Medicine Review* 1996;1:176–184.

15. Inositol hexaniacinate. *Alternative Medicine Review* 1998;3:222–223.

16. Sinatra, S. "Statins: grossly overprescribed for cholesterol and underprescribed for internal inflammation." *The Sinatra Health Report*, Sept. 2002;8:1.

17. Gouni-Berthold, I., Berthold, H.K. "Policosanol: clinical pharmacology and therapeutic significance of a new lipid-lowering agent." *American Heart Journal* 2002;143:356–365.

18. Pons, P., Mas, R., Illnait, J., et al. "Efficacy and safety of policosanol in patients with primary hypercholesterolemia." *Current Therapeutics and Research* 1992;52:507–513.

19. Aneros, E., Mas, R., Calderon, B., et al. "Effect of policosanol in lowering cholesterol levels in patients with type 2 hypercholesterolemia." *Current Therapeutics and Research* 1995;56:176–182.

20. Aneros, E., Calderon, B., Mas, R., et al. "Effect of successive dose increases of policosanol on the lipid profile and tolerability of treatment." *Current Therapeutics and Research* 1993:54:304–312.

21. Castano, G., Mas, R., Fernandez, L., et al. "Effects of policosanol 20 versus 40 mg/day in the treatment of patients with type II hypercholesterolemia: a 6-month double-blind study." *International Journal Of Clinical Pharmacologic Research* 2001;21:43–57.

22. Ortensi, G., Gladstein, J., Valli, H., et al. "A comparative study of policosanol versus simvastatin in elderly patients with hypercholesterolemia." *Current Therapeutics and Research* 1997;58:390–401.

23. Castano, G., Mas, R., Fernandez, L., et al. "Efficacy and tolerability of policosanol compared with lovastatin in patients with type 2 hypercholesterolemia and concomitant coronary risk factors." *Current Therapeutics and Research* 2000;61:137–146.

24. Janikula, M. "Policosanol: a new treatment for cardiovascular disease?" *Alternative Medicine Review* 2002;7:203–217.

25. Chagan, L., Ioselovich, A., Asherova, L., Cheng, J.W. "Use of alternative pharmacotherapy in management of cardiovascular diseases." *American Journal of Managed Care* 2002;8(3):270–285.

26. Lichtenstein, A.H. "Plant sterols and blood lipid levels." *Current Opinion in Clinical Nutrition and Metabolic Care* 2002;5(2):147–152.

27. Moghadasian, M.H., Frohlich, J.J. "Effects of dietary phytosterols on cholesterol metabolism and atherosclerosis: clinical and experimental evidence." *American Journal of Medicine* 1999;107:588–594.

28. Kerckhoffs, D.A., Brouns, F., Hornstra, G., Mensink, R.P. "Effects on the human serum lipoprotein profile of beta-glucan, soy protein and isoflavones, plant sterols and stanols, garlic and tocotrienols." *Journal of Nutrition* 2002;132(9):2494–2505.

29. Nestelss P.J. "Adulthood treatment: Cholesterol-lowering with plant sterols." *Medical Journal of Australia* 2002;176(11 Suppl):S122. Abstract.

30. Lupton, J.R., Turner, N.D. "Dietary fiber and coronary disease: does the evidence support an association." *Current Atherosclerosis Report* 2003;5:500–505.

31. Weil, A. Cardiovascular disease, June 6, 2003:www.drweil.com.

32. Singh, R.B., Niaz, M.A., Ghosh, S. "Hypolipidemic and antioxidant effects of commiphora mukul as an adjunct to dietary therapy in patients with hypercholesterolemia." *Cardiovascular Drugs and Therapeutics* 1994;8:659–664.

33. Nityanand, S., Srivastava, J.S., Asthana, O.P. "Clinical trials of guggulipid." *Journal of the Association of Physicians of India* 1990;37:323–328.

34. Szapary, P.O., Wolfe, M.L., Bloedon, L.T., et al. "Guggulipid for the treatment of hypercholesterolemia: a randomized controlled trial." *JAMA* 2003;290:765–772.

35. Maugh, T.H. "Herbal extract is faulted in study." *Los Angeles Times*, Aug. 13, 2003:A9.

36. Szapary, P.O. Personal correspondence, 12/1/03.

37. Silagy, C., Neil, A. "Garlic as a lipid lowering agent—a meta-analysis." *Journal of the Royal College of Physicians London* 1994;28:39–45.

38. Gardner, C.D., Chatterjee, L.M., Carlson, J.J. "The effect of a garlic preparation on plasma lipid levels in moderately hypercholesterolemic adults." *Atherosclerosis* 2001;154:213–220.

39. Steiner, M., Khan, A.H., Holbert, D., Lin, R.I. "A double-blind crossover study in moderately hypercholesterolemic men that compared the effect of aged garlic extract and placebo ministrations on blood lipids." *American Journal of Clinical Nutrition* 1996;64:866–870.

40. Stevinson, C., Pittler, M.H., Ernst, E. "Garlic for treating hypercholesterolemic. A meta-analysis of randomized clinical trials." *Annals of Internal Medicine* 2000;133:420–429.

41. Whitaker, J. Treatments for elevated cholesterol, 2002:www.DrWhitaker.com.

42. Food and Drug Administration. Food labeling: health claims; soy protein and coronary heart disease. 21 CFR Part 101. *Federal Register* 1999;64:57700–57733.

43. Clarkson, T.B. "Soy, soy phytoestrogens and cardiovascular disease." *Journal of Nutrition* 2002;132:566S-569S.

44. Tonstad, S., Smerud, K., Hoie, L. "The comparison of the effects of 2 doses of soy protein or casein on serum lipids, serum lipoproteins, and plasma total homocysteine in hypercholesterolemic subjects." *American Journal of Clinical Nutrition* 2002;76:78–84.

45. Desroches, S., Mauger, J.F., Ausman, L.M., et al. "Soy protein favorably affects LDL size independently of isoflavones in hypercholesterolemic men and women." *Journal of Nutrition* 2004;134:574–579.

46. Sheehan, D., Doerge, D. Letter to the Food and Drug Administration, Department of Health and Human Services. Feb. 18, 1999.

47. Mercola, J. Chemical in soybeans causes sexual dysfunctions in male rats. *eHealthy News You Can Use*, Mar. 26, 2003:www.mercola.com.

48. Whitaker, J. *Natural healing: what you're not being told.* Potomac, MD: Phillips Health, 2002.

49. "Soy: cutting through the confusion." *Consumer Reports*, July 2004:28–31.

50. Foreman, J. "Taking a closer look at soy." *Los Angeles Times*, June 14, 2004:F1.

51. Pratt, S., Matthews. C. *Super Foods.* New York: Harper Collins Publishers, Inc., 2004.

Chapter 9

1. Siguel, E.N. *Essential Fatty Acids in Health and Disease.* Brookline, MA: Nutrek Press, 1994.

2. O'Keefe, J.H. Jr, Harris, W.S. "From Inuit to implementation: omega-3 fatty acids come of age." *Mayo Clinic Proceedings* 2000;75(6):607–614.

3. "Dietary supplementation with n-3 polyunsaturated fatty acids and vitamin E after myocardial infarction: results of the GISSI-Prevenzione trial." *Lancet* 1999;354(9177):447–455.

4. de Lorgeril, M., et al. "Dietary prevention of sudden cardiac death." *European Heart Journal* 2002;23:277–285.

5. Albert, C.M., et al. "Blood levels of long-chain N-3 fatty acids and the risk of sudden death." *The New England Journal of Medicine* 2002;346(15):1113–1118.

6. Hu, F.B., et al. "Fish and omega-3 fatty acid intake and risk of coronary heart disease in women." *JAMA* 2002;287(14):1815–1821.

7. Marchioli, R., et al. "Early protection against sudden death by N-3 polyunsaturated fatty acids after myocardial infarction." *Circulation* 2002;105:1897–1903.

8. Renaud, S.C., Lanzmann-Petithory, D. "Coronary heart disease: dietary links and pathogeneisis." *Public Health and Nutrition* 2001:459–474.

9. Simopoulos, A.P. "Essential fatty acids in health and chronic disease." *American Journal of Clinical Nutrition* 1999;70(suppl):560S-569S.

10. Demaison, L., Moreau, D. *Cellular and Molecular Life Science* 2002;59:463–477.

11. Sinatra, S. *Coenzyme* Q_{10}, Sept. 26 2002:http://www.drsinatra.com/index.asp.

12. Brody, J.E. "Tip the scale in favor of fish: the healthful benefits await." *The New York Times*, July 29, 2003:nytimes.com.

13. Weil, A. Cardiovascular disease, June 6, 2003:www.drweil.com.

14. Sinatra, S. Health Email Reoprt, 8/21/03.

15. Mercury in seafood linked to infertility. *Reuters Health,* Sept. 24, 2002: www.reuters.com.

16. Mercola, J. Mercury in fish. www.mercola.com/2002/jun/5/toxic_waste.htm:3/3/2003.

17. Whitaker, J. *Sidestep Your Side Effects.* Potomac, MD: Phillips Health, 2002.

18. Wright, K. "B-vitamin linked to healthy hearts." *San Diego Union-Tribune,* 1/19/02:E1.

19. McCully, K.S. "Homocysteine, folate, vitamin B6, and cardiovascular disease." *JAMA* 1998;280:417.

20. Bazzano, L.A., He, J., Ogden, L.G., et al. "Dietary intake of folate and risk of stroke in U.S. men and women: NHANES I epidemiologic follow-up study." *Stroke* 2002;33:1183–1189.

21. Hackam, D.G., Peterson, J.C., Spence, J.D. "What level of plasma homocysteine should be treated? Effects of vitamin therapy on progression of carotid atherosclerosis in patients with homocysteine levels above and below 14 micromoles/L." *American Journal of Hypertension* 2000;13(1 Pt1):105–110.

22. Rydlewicz A., Simpson J.A., Taylor R.J., et al. "The effect of folic acid supplementation on plasma homocysteine in an elderly population." *QJM* 2002;95(1):27–35.

23. Hirschenbein, N. Personal communication, June 10, 2003.

24. Kannel, W.B. Cardioprotection: What is it? Who needs it? *Protection across the Cardiovascular Continuum,* University of Cincinnati 2002:4–11.

25. *Facts about Dietary Supplements.* Office of Dietary Supplements, National Institutes of Health, Mar. 2001.

26. Topalov, V., Kovacevic, D., Topalov, A., et al. "Magnesium in cardiology." *Medicinski Pregled* [Medical Review (Croatian)] 2000;53:319–324, Abstract.

27. Carper, J. Mighty magnesium: This overlooked nutrient fights against heart disease, pain and diabetes. *USA Weekend,* Aug. 30, 2002:http://usaweekend.com.

28. Oladapo, O.O., *African Journal of Medicine and Medical Science* 2000;29:265–268.

29. Wright, J.V. *Nutrition & Healing,* March 2003:4.

30. Sinatra, S. *2003 Consumer's Guide to Rx and OTC Drugs.* Potomac, MD: Phillips Health, 2003.

31. Rakel, R.E. *Conn's Current Therapy.* Philadelphia: W.B. Saunders Company, 1993.

Chapter 10

1. *Physicians' Desk Reference,* 57th edition. Montvale, NJ: Medical Economics Company, 2003.

2. *American Hospital Formulary Service, Drug Information 2002.* Gerald K. McEvoy, editor. Bethesda, MD: American Society of Hospital Pharmacists. 2002.

3. Haney, D.Q. (Associated Press). "Study finds Atkins diet may have surprising benefit on cholesterol." *San Diego Union-Tribune,* November 18, 2002.

4. Roberts, W.C. "Preventing and arresting coronary atherosclerosis." *American Heart Journal* 1995;130(3 Pt 1):580–600.

5. Noonan, D. "You want statins with that?" *Newsweek* 7/14/O3:48–53.

6. Johnston, C.S., Tjonn, S.L., Swan, P.D. "High-protein, low-fat diets are effective for weight loss and favorably alter biomarkers in healthy adults." *Journal of Nutrition* 2004;134:586–591.

7. Patrick, L., Uzick, M. "Cardiovascular disease: C-reactive protein and the inflammatory disease paradigm." *Alternative Medicine Review* 2001;6:248–271.

8. Trichopoulou, A., Costacou, T., Bamia, C., Trichopoulos, D. "Adherence to a Mediterranean diet and survival in a Greek population." *The New England Journal of Medicine* 2003;348:2599–2608.

9. Willett, W.C. *Mediterranean Diet and Health.* Pages 24–26 in The Best of Experts Speak. Sacramento, ITServices: 2000.

10. Esselstyn, C.B. *Becoming Heart Attack Proof.* Cleveland Clinic Foundation: www.heart attackproof.com.

11. Ornish, D., Scherwitz, L.W., Billings, J.H., et al. "Intensive lifestyle changes for reversal of coronary heart disease." *JAMA* 1998;280(23):2001–2007.

12. Ornish D. "Avoiding revascularization with lifestyle changes: The Multicenter Lifestyle Demonstration Project." *American Journal of Cardiology* 1998;82(10B):72T–76T.

13. Lakka, H., Laakosonen, D.E., Lakka, T.A., et al. "The metabolic syndrome and total and cardiovascular disease mortality in middle-aged men." *JAMA* 2002;288:2709–2716.

14. Wright, J. "Should you go low-carb?" *Nutrition & Healing,* June 2004;11:1–5.

15. Park, Y.W., et al. "The metabolic syndrome: prevalence and associated risk factor findings in the US population from the Third National Health and Nutrition Examination Survey, 1988–1994." *Archives of Internal Medicine* 2003;163:427–436.

16. Ford, E.S., Giles, W.H., Dietz, W.H. "Prevalence of the metabolic syndrome in U.S. adults: findings from NHANES III." *JAMA* 2002;287:356–359.

17. Hoffman, R. Personal communication, July 18, 2004.

18. Baker, J. Personal communication, July 1, 2002.

19. Bravata, D.M., Sanders, L.S., Huang, J., et al. "Efficacy and safety of low-carbohydrate diet." *JAMA* 2003;289:1837–1850.

20. Foster, G.D., et al. "A Randomized Trial of a Low-Carbohydrate Diet for Obesity." *The New England Journal of Medicine* 2003;348:2082–2092.

21. The Diet That Works. *The Wall Street Journal,* April 22, 2003:www.wsj.com.

22. Brody, J.E. "Fear not that carrot, potato, or ear of corn." *The New York Times,* June 11, 2002.

23. Mirkin, G. *Glycemic Load,* 11/15/01:www.drmirkin.com/nutrition/9566.html.

24. Liu, S. "Intake of refined carbohydrates and whole grain foods in relation to risk of type 2 diabetes mellitus and coronary heart disease." *Journal of the American College of Nutrition* 2002;21(4):298–306.

25. Willett W., Manson J., Liu S. "Glycemic index, glycemic load, and risk of type 2 diabetes." *American Journal of Clinical Nutrition* 2002;76(1):274S–280S.

26. Hallfrisch J., Behall, K.M. "Mechanisms of the effects of grains on insulin and glucose responses." *American Journal of Clinical Nutrition* 2000;19(3 Suppl):320S–325S.

27. Liu, S. "Whole-grain foods, dietary fiber, and type 2 diabetes: searching for a kernel of truth." *American Journal of Clinical Nutrition* 2003;77:527–529.

28. Liu, S., Manson, J.E., Stampfer, M.J., et al. "A prospective study of whole-grain and risk of type 2 diabetes mellitus in US women." *American Journal of Public Health* 2000; 90(9):1409–1415.

29. Slavin, J.L. "Mechanisms for the impact of whole grain foods on cancer risk." *Journal of the American College of Nutrition* 2000;19(3 Suppl):300S–307S.

30. La Vecchia, C., Chataenod, L., Altieri, A., Tavani, A. "Nutrition and health: epidemiology of diet, cancer and cardiovascular disease in Italy." *Nutrition and Metabolism in Cardiovascular Disease* 2001;11(4 Suppl):10–15.

31. Liu, S., Sesso, H.D., Manson, J.E., et al. "Is intake of breakfast cereals related to total and cause-specific mortality in men?" *American Journal of Clinical Nutrition* 2003;77:594–599.

32. Periera, M.A., Jacobs, D.R., Pins, J.J., et al. "Effect of whole grains on insulin sensitivity in overweight hyperinsulinemic adults." *American Journal of Clinical Nutrition* 2000;75:848–55.

33. Brody, J.E. For unrefined healthfulness: whole grains. *The New York Times,* Mar. 4, 2003:www.nytimes.com.

34. Tufts University Health & Nutrition Letter, June 2003:21:8.

35. Hu, F.B., Willett, W.C. "Optimal diets for prevention of coronary heart disease." *JAMA* 2002;288:2569–2578.

36. Wolcott, W.L. *The Metabolic Typing Diet.* New York: Doubleday, 2000.

37. Wolcott, W.L. Metabolic typing. eHealthy News You Can Use e-newsletter, Dec. 18, 2002;386:www.mercola.com.

38. Hellmich, N., Rubin, R. "Health guidelines: It's tough keeping up." *USA Today,* June 16, 2003:1A.

36. Liu, S., Manson, J.E., Stampfer, M.J., et al. "A prospective study of whole-grain intake and risk of type 2 diabetes mellitus in US women." *American Journal of Public Health* 2000;90(9):1409–1415.

37. Slavin, J.L. "Mechanisms for the impact of whole grain foods on cancer risk." *Journal of the American College of Nutrition* 2000;19(3 Suppl):300S–307S.

38. La Vecchia, C., Chatenoud, L., Altieri, A., Tavani, A. "Nutrition and health: epidemiology of diet, cancer and cardiovascular disease in Italy." *Nutrition and Metabolism in Cardiovascular Disease* 2001;11(4 Suppl):10–15.

Chapter 11

1. Winslow, B., McGinley, L., Adams, C. "States, Insurers Find Prescriptions for High Drug Costs." *The Wall Street Journal*, Sept. 11, 2002:A1,8.

Conclusion

1. Jackevicius, C.A., Mamdani, M., Tu, J.V. "Adherence with statin therapy in elderly patients with and without acute coronary syndromes." *JAMA* 2002;288:462–467.

2. Benner, J.S., Glynn, R.J., Mogun, H., et al. "Long-term persistence in use of statin therapy in elderly patients." *JAMA* 2002;288:455–461.

3. Parker-Pope, T. "Breakthrough! Ten major medical advances you're likely to see in the coming year." *The Wall Street Journal* January 26, 2004:R1.

4. Gilroy, C.M., Steiner, J.F., Byers, T.B., et al. "Echinacea and truth in labeling." *Archives of Internal Medicine* 2003;163:699–704.

5. Jenkins, D.J., Kendall, C.W., Marchie, A., et al. "Effects of a dietary portfolio of cholesterol-lowering foods vs. lovastatin on serum lipids and C-reactive protein." JAMA 2003;290:502–509.

6. Sylvester, B. "Ape diet" equals cholesterol drugs. UPI Science News, 7/25/2003.

7. Anderson, J.W. "Diet first, then medication for hypercholesterolemia." JAMA 2003;290:531–533.

8. American Medical Association Council on Ethical and Judicial Affairs. *Code of Medical Ethics*, 1998–1999 edition. Chicago, IL: American Medical Association, 1997.

About the Author

Dr. Jay Cohen is a widely recognized expert on prescription medications and non-drug alternatives that work. Dr. Cohen is an Associate Professor (voluntary) of Family and Preventive Medicine and of Psychiatry at the University of California, San Diego. Dr. Cohen is also the Chairman of the Medical Advisory Committee of The Erythromelalgia Association.

Dr. Cohen graduated cum laude and the equivalent of Phi Beta Kappa from Ursinus College in 1967. He earned his medical degree at Temple University in 1971. After completing his internship, Dr. Cohen practiced general medicine, then conducted pain research at UCLA. He then completed a psychiatry residency at the University of California, San Diego, and practiced psychiatry and psychopharmacology until 1990.

Since 1990, Dr. Cohen has been conducting independent research on the causes of medication side effects, while seeking solutions to solve this decades-long problem. Dr. Cohen has published his findings in leading medical journals including *Archives of Internal Medicine, The Journal of the American Medical Women's Association, Geriatrics, Drug Safety,* and the *Annals of Pharmacotherapy.* He has also written articles for consumer publications such as *Newsweek, Bottom Line Health,* and *Life Extension Magazine.* His work has been featured in numerous magazines and newspapers including *The New York Times, Washington Post, Consumer Reports, The Wall Street Journal, Modern Maturity, Women's Day.* His book, *Over Dose: The Case Against The Drug Companies* (Tarcher/Putnam, 2001), received unanimously excellent reviews from *Publishers Weekly, Library Journal,* and others, as well as in the *Journal of the American Medical Association.*

Dr. Cohen has been featured on more than seventy-five radio programs across America, including the "People's Pharmacy" and National Public

Radio's "Morning Edition." Dr. Cohen has spoken at conferences of patients, doctors, drug industry executives, and malpractice attorneys. In October 2001, during the anthrax scare, Dr. Cohen's article on severe reactions to Cipro, Levaquin, and other fluoroquinolone antibiotics triggered a national debate on the best treatment for anthrax and prompted the U.S. Centers for Disease Control to alter their treatment guidelines. In November 2002, Dr. Cohen was the keynote speaker at the Annual Science Day of the U.S. Food and Drug Administration's Clinical Pharmacology Division. He has also debated Dr. Robert Temple, the FDA's top drug expert, on multiple occasions, most recently at the March 2004 meeting of the American Society for Clinical Pharmacology and Therapeutics.

Dr. Cohen has never accepted funding from the drug industry. Dr. Cohen conducts his research and writing in Del Mar, California.

INDEX

Cytochrome 2D6 (CYP2D6), 65, 67
Cytochrome 3A4 (CYP3A4), 67
Cytochrome P450 enzymes, 65–66,
    68, 69

D
Derealization, 90
Diets
    choosing healthy, 132–133,
        144–147
    low-carbohydrate, 136–140
    low-fat, 133–136
    of whole grains, 140–144
Doerge, Daniel, 116
Drugs, metabolizing of, 65–68

E
Ehrlich, Robert, 37
Erythromelalgia, 129
Esselstyn, Caldwell, 135
Essential fatty acids.
    See Omega-3 fatty acids.
Every-other-day approach, 55, 153
Exercise, 147–148
Extensive metabolizers (EM), 65, 69

F
Fiber, 112
Fibrinogen, 30
First-dose reactions, 40, 90–91
First-dose reactivity, 40
Fish oils. *See* Omega-3 fatty acids.
Folic acid, 29–30, 126–127
Furberg, Curt, 44

G
Ganiats, Ted, 32
Garlic, 114–115
General medication sensitivity,
    68–69, 70–72

Glycemic index, 140
Glycemic load, 140
Golomb, Beatrice, 87
Graham, David, 44
Grains, 140–144
Grapefruit juice, 67
Graveline, Duane, 15, 16, 77, 87
Guarneri, Mimi, 127
Guggulipid, 112–114
Guggulsterone, 112
Gum guggul. *See* Guggulipid.
Gurwitz, Jerry, 83

H
HDL-C. *See* High-density
    lipoprotein cholesterol.
Heber, David, 103
Hendler, Sheldon, 74
Herxheimer, Andrew, 36, 82, 92
High-density lipoprotein
    cholesterol (HDL-C), 21–22
Hirschenbein, Neil, 127
Hoffman, Ron, 137
Homocysteine, 29, 105, 126, 127
Horton, Richard, 44
Hu, Frank, 145
Hypertension, 129

I
Individual variation, 14–15
Inflammation, 26, 122, 124
Inositol hexaniacinate, 106–108, 155
Inter-individual variation, 15
Intermediate metabolizers (IM),
    65, 69
Interstitial pulmonary fibrosis,
    93, 94

K
Kessler, David, 88

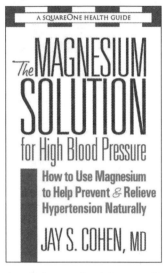

A SQUAREONE HEALTH GUIDE

The MAGNESIUM SOLUTION for High Blood Pressure

How to Use Magnesium to Help Prevent & Relieve Hypertension Naturally

JAY S. COHEN, MD

THE MAGNESIUM SOLUTION FOR HIGH BLOOD PRESSURE

How to Use Magnesium to Help Prevent and Relieve Hypertension Naturally

Jay S. Cohen, MD

Approximately 23 percent of all Americans have hypertension, more commonly known as high blood pressure. Without proper treatment, hypertension can lead to hardening of the arteries, heart attack, and stroke. Unfortunately, the conventional medicines used to treat this condition come with potentially dangerous side effects. When Dr. Jay Cohen—physician, medical researcher, and professor of medicine—learned of his own vascular condition, he was well aware of the risks associated with the standard treatments. Based upon his research, he selected a safer drug-free option—magnesium.

The Magnesium Solution for High Blood Pressure is a direct result of Dr. Cohen's experience. It is a concise easy-to-understand guide that explains what hypertension is, what magnesium is, and the key role magnesium plays in preventing and treating this condition. The book carefully describes the most effective types of magnesium for treating hypertension; how magnesium interacts with diuretics and blood pressure drugs; and how much magnesium to take. It also details how to use magnesium in conjunction with hypertension meds. All of the information is backed by relevant scientific studies and interviews with leading experts in the field.

For those who are looking for a safe, effective, natural approach to the treatment of high blood pressure, Dr. Cohen prescribes a proven natural remedy in *The Magnesium Solution for High Blood Pressure*.

ABOUT THE AUTHOR

Jay S. Cohen, MD, is an Associate Professor (voluntary) of Family and Preventive Medicine and of Psychiatry at the University of California, San Diego. He has published numerous research articles, as well as articles in *Newsweek, Life Extension magazine,* and *Bottom Line Health,* and is also the author of *Over Dose: The Case Against the Drug Companies.* Dr. Cohen and his family live in Del Mar, California.

$5.95 • 96 pages • 4 x 7.5-inch paperback • ISBN 0-7570-0255-2

THE MAGNESIUM SOLUTION FOR MIGRAINE HEADACHES

How to Use Magnesium to Prevent and Relieve Migraine and Cluster Headaches Naturally

Jay S. Cohen, MD

Over 30 million people across North America suffer from migraine headaches. Some use medications to dull the ache, while others choose to simply bear the pain. Over the years, a number of drugs have been developed to treat migraines; however, these treatments don't work for everyone. Furthermore, they come with a high risk of dangerous side effects. Fortunately, Dr. Jay S. Cohen—physician, medical researcher, and professor of medicine—has discovered an alternative. Magnesium, an effective drug-free option, offers a proven way to not only prevent migraines, but also stop them in their tracks.

The Magnesium Solution for Migraine Headaches is a direct result of Dr. Cohen's research. This concise easy-to-understand guide explains what a migraine is; details how magnesium relaxes the nerves and blood vessels involved in migraines; and shows how this supplement can play a key role in preventing and treating migraine headaches. The book also describes why magnesium is as effective as drugs, as well as safer and less expensive; what type of magnesium works best; and how much magnesium should be taken to prevent or stop migraines. All of the information is backed by relevant scientific studies and interviews with leading experts in the field.

For those who are looking for a safe and effective approach to the prevention and treatment of migraine and cluster headaches Dr. Cohen prescribes a proven natural remedy in *The Magnesium Solution for Migraine Headaches*.

$5.95 • 96 pages • 4 x 7.5-inch paperback• ISBN 0-7570-0256-0

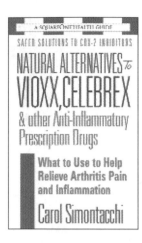

Natural Alternatives to Vioxx, Celebrex & Other Anti-Inflammatory Prescription Drugs

What to Use To Help Relieve Arthritis Pain and Inflammation

Carol Simontacchi, CCN, MS

Beyond today's headlines and pharmaceutical spin is an underlying truth—COX-2 inhibitor drugs can be extremely dangerous to your health. While this class of drugs does relieve pain and inflammation, the potential for heart attack and stroke has proven too great a risk for many. For those who are now looking for other options, health expert Carol Simontacchi has put together a simple guide to using safer natural alternatives. Written in easy-to-understand language, here is a book that provides solid information about nature's most effective treatments.

The book begins by examining the causes of arthritis pain and inflammation. It looks first at the pharmaceutical approach to dealing with this condition, and then at the holistic approach. This is followed by a concise discussion of the most effective natural supplements available, including curcumin, cat's claw, fish oil, ginger root, glucosamine, chondroitin, MSM, and SierraSil. Each supplement is examined for its method of action, scientific documentation, and proper dosage. Important information is included on identifying the best natural products.

Clearly, there is a place for drugs, but becoming a human guinea pig should not be part of the equation. Although natural product companies may not have the advertising dollars enjoyed by the pharmaceutical industry, the beneficial effects of natural remedies should not be overlooked. *Natural Alternatives to Vioxx, Celebrex & Other Anti-Inflammatory Prescription Drugs* provides a vital resource for those looking for a safer solution.

ABOUT THE AUTHOR

Carol Simontacchi, CCN, MS, is a certified clinical nutritionist and the author of a number of books on nutrition, including *Your Fat Is Not Your Fault, The Crazy Makers, A Woman's Guide to a Healthy Heart ,* and *Weight Success for A Lifetime.* In addition, Ms. Simontacchi is a highly sought-after lecturer who speaks to professional and lay audiences across the country on important health topics. She has appeared on numerous national, regional, and local radio and TV shows, and her work has been featured in *Newsday, First for Women, Women's Day,* and other popular publications. Ms. Simontacchi currently lives with her family in Florida.

$5.95 • 96 pages • 4 x 7.5-inch paperback • ISBN 0-7570-0278-1

ULCER FREE!

Nature's Safe and Effective Remedy for Ulcers

Georges M. Halpern, MD, PhD

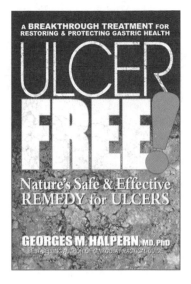

Approximately 4 million Americans are annually diagnosed with peptic ulcer disease. The resulting gastritis—inflammation of the stomach—causes heartburn, nausea, gas, reflux, and stomach pain. For years, standard treatment consisted of antacids to relieve symptoms, dietary changes, and, in some cases, operations designed to freeze the affected areas of the stomach. Later, when it was discovered that ulcers were actually caused by a bacterium, antibiotics became the treatment of choice. While more effective than previous attempts at relief, this cure came with its own set of risks, ranging from often severe side effects to drug-resistant bacterial strains. For many, the treatment's problems outweighed its benefits.

Now, a major breakthrough in nutritional science offers a safe, simple, and totally natural approach to treating this gastric problem. *Ulcer Free!* is the remarkable story of zinc-carnosine, a new dietary supplement that has been proven to heal ulcers and relieve symptoms. Here, you'll learn of its discovery, its ten years of clinical studies as an alternative therapy, and its US patent approval. Just as important, you'll learn how this new supplement can be used to successfully treat ulcer pain.

If you or a loved one suffers from ulcers, you know that the cure can sometimes be as bad as the problem. In *Ulcer Free!*, you'll discover how zinc-carnosine is offering a safe cure to millions of ulcer sufferers.

ABOUT THE AUTHOR

Georges M. Halpern, MD, PhD, attended medical school at the University of Paris, France. He subsequently received a PhD from the Faculty of Pharmacy, University of Paris XI—Chatenay Malabry. A Fellow of the American Academy of Allergy and Immunology, Dr. Halpern is board certified in internal medicine and allergy, and is Professor Emeritus of Medicine at the University of California—Davis. He is also a Distinguished Professor of Medicine at the University of Hong Kong. The author resides in Portola Valley, California.

$14.95 • 176 pages • 6 x 9-inch paperback • ISBN 0-7570-0253-6

Relieving Pain Naturally

Safe and Effective Alternative Approaches To Treating and Overcoming Chronic Illness

Sylvia Goldfarb, PhD and Roberta W. Waddell

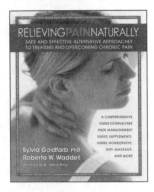

For millions of Americans, severe pain is a fact of everyday life. Standard medicine commonly offers relief through drug therapies. While often effective, these medications come with a host of side effects— disorientation, drowsiness, mental impairment, nausea, peptic ulcers, tinnitus, and addiction, to mention just a few. Moreover, after prolonged use, the body's tolerance to many of these drugs requires increased dosages to remain effective. While many sufferers would prefer nondrug options, much of the available information on alternative pain treatment is scattered, incomplete, self-serving, and in many instances, out of date—or it was, until now. Professional health writers Dr. Sylvia Goldfarb and Roberta Waddell have designed *Relieving Pain Naturally* to be a comprehensive guide to drug-free pain management. Here is an up-to-date resource that is written in clear nontechnical language for ease of use and quick accessibility.

Relieving Pain Naturally is divided into two parts. Part One examines over forty of the most common chronic pain-related conditions, from abdominal pain to sciatica to tendonitis. Each disorder is explained, and its alternative pain treatments detailed. Part Two offers twenty-seven drug-free therapies. These entries include both conventional treatments and alternative modalities such as acupuncture, biofeedback, heat and cold therapy, hypnosis, nutrition, and oxygen therapy. Also included are clinical studies and cautions, where applicable. A comprehensive resource guide provides a list of groups and professional organizations that can help you find the appropriate therapist in your area.

For years, millions of pain sufferers have longed for a safe, side effect-free treatment for chronic pain, but have been unsure how to take that first step towards greater health. Now, *Relieving Pain Naturally* provides a reliable starting point.

ABOUT THE AUTHORS

Sylvia Goldfarb, PhD, a writer specializing in medical topics, has written articles for numerous magazines, including *Focus, Natural Body and Fitness,* and *Today's O.R. Nurse.* She is also the author of two books, including *Allergy Relief.* Dr. Goldfarb resides in Philadelphia, Pennsylvania.

Roberta W. Waddell has been both a writer and editor in the field of alternative health for over sixteen years. Because of her own chronic pain, she has experienced conventional and alternative therapies firsthand.

$18.95 • 320 pages • 8.5 x 11-inch paperback • ISBN 0-7570-0079-7

STOPPING INFLAMMATION

Relieving the Cause of Degenerative Diseases

Nancy Appleton, PhD

Inflammation is a word we hear all the time— *"Your throat is inflamed," "You have some inflammation around the knee," "You have an inflamed ear."* Most of us think of it as a symptom associated with an infection, irritation, or injury. Dr. Nancy Appleton, however, has discovered that it might be more than just a simple reaction to a health disorder. When the body's tissues are disturbed in some manner, a series of complex reactions takes place: the affected area draws fluid to itself, swells, heats up, and generates liquid by-products. In other words, it becomes inflamed. In most cases, when the disorder stops, the tissue returns to its normal healthy state. Sometimes, though, the tissue remains chronically inflamed. Dr. Appleton's early research demonstrated that this chronic condition might be more harmful than ever suspected. Soon, she began to ask questions: What if inflammation was at the heart of various degenerative diseases? What health benefits could be gained if we could stop inflammation? *Stopping Inflammation* is the result of Dr. Appleton's ten-year quest to answer these important questions.

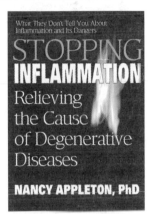

Drawing on the latest medical research, the book begins with a full explanation of inflammation. It then looks at its many causes, from food allergies to environmental factors to psychological stress. Next, it focuses on the various health disorders that afflict modern society— obesity, addiction, heart disease, diabetes, cancer, bowel disorders, and so many more—and explains the role that inflammation plays in each of these diseases. The book then provides a number of fresh non-drug treatments aimed not at controlling the problem, but at removing its cause.

Twenty years ago, Dr. Nancy Appleton's groundbreaking bestseller *Lick the Sugar Habit* exposed the dangers of ingesting excessive amounts of sugar. In her newest work, *Stopping Inflammation*, Dr. Appleton examines the larger picture of twenty-first-century disease, and finds the underlying cause. Just as important, she offers safe and credible solutions.

ABOUT THE AUTHOR

Nancy Appleton, PhD, earned her BS in clinical nutrition from UCLA and her PhD in health services from Walden University. She maintains a private practice in Santa Monica, California. An avid researcher, Dr. Appleton lecturers extensively throughout the world, and has appeared on numerous television and radio talk shows. She is the best-selling author of *Lick the Sugar Habit* and *Healthy Bones*.

$14.95 • 228 pages • 6 x 9-inch paperback • ISBN 0-7570-0148-3

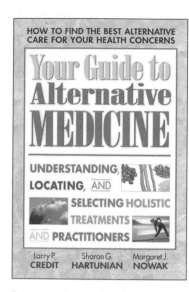

HOW TO FIND THE BEST ALTERNATIVE CARE FOR YOUR HEALTH CONCERNS

Your Guide to Alternative Medicine

Understanding, Locating, and Selecting Holistic Treatments and Practitioners

Larry P. Credit, Sharon G. Hartunian, and Margaret J. Nowak

The growing world of complementary medicine offers safe and effective solutions to many health disorders, from backache to headache. The more you know about these alternative health techniques, the greater your chance of selecting the right remedy for your own health problem. You may already be interested in some of the alternative care approaches that are attracting growing attention—for example, acupuncture, chiropractic, homeopathy, and various types of massage. But if you're like most people, you have a hundred and one questions you'd like answered before you choose a treatment. "Will I feel the acupuncture needles?" "Does chiropractic hurt?" "What is a homeopathic remedy?" "Does massage really work?" *Your Guide to Alternative Medicine* provides the fundamental facts and practical guidance necessary to choose an effective complementary care therapy and begin treatment.

This comprehensive reference clearly explains numerous approaches in an easy-to-read quick-reference format. For every complementary care option discussed, there is a description and brief history; a list of conditions that respond; information on the cost and duration of treatment; credentials and educational background for practitioners; a directory of professional organizations that can offer you further information; and more.

To find those therapies most appropriate for a specific condition, there is also a unique troubleshooting chart that lists common disorders along with the complementary approaches best suited to treat them.

Your Guide to Alternative Medicine introduces you to options that you may never have considered—methods that enhance the body's natural healing potential and have few, if any, side effects. Have you thought about using an herbal treatment to reduce allergies? Did you know that aromatherapy can relieve nausea? If you have questions about complementary health care, *Your Guide to Alternative Medicine* has the answers. Here is a reference that can help you make informed decisions about all your important healthcare needs.

$11.95 • 208 pages • 6 x 9-inch paperback • ISBN 0-7570-0125-4